T0195863

Also by Denise Tarasuk, ND

*Tics and Tourette's Syndrome: An Ayurvedic
Approach to Health and Happiness*

*Monsoon Medicine: A Diary of a Canadian
Medicine Woman & Tales of a Bengali Doctor*

*Monsoon Medicine: Homeopathy,
Keynotes & Materia Medica*

POCKET GUIDE

HOMEOPATHIC FIRST AID FOR VACCINOSIS

With Comparative Materia Medica

Denise Tarasuk, ND

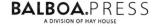
BALBOA.PRESS
A DIVISION OF HAY HOUSE

Balboa Press books may be ordered through booksellers or by contacting:

Balboa Press
A Division of Hay House
1663 Liberty Drive
Bloomington, IN 47403
www.balboapress.com
844-682-1282

Because of the dynamic nature of the Internet, any web addresses or
links contained in this book may have changed since publication and
may no longer be valid. The views expressed in this work are solely those
of the author and do not necessarily reflect the views of the publisher,
and the publisher hereby disclaims any responsibility for them.

The author of this book does not dispense medical advice or prescribe the use
of any technique as a form of treatment for physical, emotional, or medical
problems without the advice of a physician, either directly or indirectly. The
intent of the author is only to offer information of a general nature to help
you in your quest for emotional and spiritual well-being. In the event you use
any of the information in this book for yourself, which is your constitutional
right, the author and the publisher assume no responsibility for your actions.

Print information available on the last page.

ISBN: 979-8-7652-2980-4 (sc)
ISBN: 979-8-7652-2981-1 (e)

Library of Congress Control Number: 2022910946

Balboa Press rev. date: 07/21/2022

Dedication

This book is dedicated to my loving husband, Matthew Tarasuk, who is always at the right place at the right time. His support is beyond description and that makes him absolutely perfect.

On Children

And a woman who held a babe against her bosom said,
Speak to us of Children.
And he said:
Your children are not your children.
They are the sons and daughters of Life's longing for itself.
They come through you but not from you,
And though they are with you yet they belong not to you,

You may give them your love but not your thoughts.
For they have their own thoughts.
You may house their bodies but not their souls,
For their souls dwell in the house of tomorrow, which
you cannot visit, not even in your dreams.

You may strive to be like them, but seek not to make
them like you.
For life goes not backward nor tarries with yesterday.
You are the bows from which your children as living
arrows are sent forth.
The archer sees the mark upon the path of the infinite,
and He
bends you with His might that His arrows may go swift
and far.
Let your bending in the archer's hand be for gladness;
For even as He loves the arrow that flies, so He loves
also the bow that is stable.

The Prophet, Kahlil Gibran
Knopf, 1923

Contents

Foreword

It is essential in this day and age, due to the widespread obsession with instant access and success, to get back to the basics of homeopathy. I applaud Dr. Tarasuk, for that is exactly what she has done here in *Pocket Guide: Homeopathic First-Aid for Vaccinosis.* Dr. Tarasuk's writing is lucid, easy to understand, and expressed with her unique warmth and compassion, illustrating so clearly her commitment to place the patient above all else.

Dr. Tarasuk has followed in my footsteps with patient care and now to my delight, she has written her own Materia Medica! With keynotes and a touch of humor, the reader will find it easy and pleasing to remember the remedies. She has taken my teaching and turned these teachings into practical and healing words.

To practice at such a deep level of homeopathy is very rare. This art is two-fold and takes years to learn. First, one must understand the efficacy of each remedy, and second, correctly utilize the science of Comparative Materia Medica to select the optimal remedy.

The art of Materia Medica is almost lost. These twelve remedies, along with Comparative Materia Medica, represent the key to solving the puzzling and often painful experience of Vaccinosis. Parents rejoice! It is my hope that this guide will lead the way to restore other works from the great masters and bring alive the principles of homeopathy.

This book brings me great joy. No doubt, with a bit of study, our readers will be excited and find the remedies easy to learn. To close, I say good luck and always be a good student. Time is so precious, so with each day, read a little homeopathy. You will become a great prescriber.

Dr. Sunirmal Sarkar, MD, PhD

Introduction

The idea for a homeopathic book on Vaccinosis grew out of my annual lecture at the Autism One Conference. Each year I presented a remedy that had a significant impact on children's development and health. In 2007, my topic was Thuja occidentalis, "The Tree of Life."

Several homeopaths approached me afterward saying they had never heard of the remedy or were unfamiliar with its use. I was indeed surprised as Thuja is considered a polycrest, a drug that serves as a remedy for many diseases and is essential when there is a history of vaccinosis.

Shortly after the conference, seeing the need to fill in the gap that existed, I wrote a 150-page treatise on Thuja occidentalis. I also continued to explore and document my clinical findings and observations regarding the use of various remedies on the children I treated in my practice.

The *Pocket Guide: Homeopathic First-Aid for Vaccinosis* is a guide with 12 selected remedies and Comparative Materia Medica. The guide, designed for use as an easy reference and desk-side companion, contains the foremost remedies for the patient who suffers from side effects or presents with a history of vaccinosis.

Keynotes and Case Studies

This handbook is unique. Though a brief treatise, its pages pull together historical, practical, and contemporary evidence-based clinical experience to help you learn and effectively treat patients who suffer from the bad effect of vaccination as the result of the widespread and recent worldwide pandemic. The information offered here is based on my own case studies and clinical experience. I have relied on Dr. Sunirmal Sarkar's knowledge and wisdom as well, and most importantly, on the literature of the Grand Masters.

The beginning of each chapter provides an at-a-glance overview of symptoms and characteristics that relate to the selected remedy. These Keynotes from the masters list mental and physical symptoms, ameliorations, and aggravations. Study and familiarity with these keynotes is the foundation of successful treatments.

Many of the case studies, altered for privacy, are taken from my personal practice, where I have treated many children on the autism spectrum. Other cases are taken from a patient's history when working with Dr. Sarkar in West Bengal, India. Working with Dr. Sarkar for over 20 years, a master of homeopathy and Materia Medica, has given me confidence and the opportunity to see and treat many unusual cases that would not be possible to witness in Canada or the USA.

The Grand Masters

The legacy of the Grand Masters of homeopathy is a gift to humanity and a responsibility I take seriously to make available to both the new and experienced generation of homeopaths. Their research and provings are invaluable. If we neglect their study, we are at risk of losing this precious legacy.

The experience and provings from the Grand Masters of homeopathy will assist you in understanding the remedy and applying it in a clinical case or setting. As a Naturopathic doctor, I have centered my work by reading and analyzing books left by the Grand Masters such as Dr. E. B Nash, Dr. J.C. Burnett, Dr. H.C Allen, Dr. M.L. Tyler, Dr. W. Boericke, Dr. P. Sankaran, Dr. M. Blackie, Dr. D. Borland, Dr. J. Clarke, Dr. Boger, Dr. C. Hering, Dr. C. von Boenninghausen, and Dr. N.M. Choudhuri.

The Grand Masters of homeopathy have guided my work, both as a writer and medical practice doctor. I would be lost without the Grand Masters of Homeopathy. Although their information can be complicated to understand, they have become my friends, and life without their comments would be dull indeed. I am particularly fond of Dr. E.B. Nash's writing. He has been an important influence on my writing.

Comparative Media Medica

Comparison between remedies is essential in order to make a proper treatment plan. With the clinical tips from this pocket guide, the homeopath will acquire a sound scientific approach to homeopathic prescription. For the sake of the patient, the practitioner of homeopathy must continuously think about Comparative Materia Medica, a key component of any diagnostic and treatment process.

Tribute

Throughout this book, you'll find many tributes and stories about my time with Dr. Sarkar. The value of the lessons he imparted to me cannot be exaggerated. Working alongside him year after year in a village on the outskirts of Kolkata has broadened my skill set as a physician. Seeing an unbelievable number of patients daily in his clinic introduced me to tropical diseases and sequela of diseases such as smallpox that cannot be seen in California. Using modern diagnostic tools such as blood tests, MRI, X-rays, and ultrasounds to diagnose and follow up demonstrates how solid and reliable homeopathy treatments are.

I still remember the day that Dr. Sarkar gave me a copy of his private notebook filled with clinical gems and pearls. He then stated with a solemn face, "I have written my own Materia Medica, now you must write yours!"

My wish for you, dear readers, is that you will make use of this information and pass on the wisdom of homeopathy to the next generation.

Dr. Denise Tarasuk, ND

NOTE ON INCONSISTENCIES: Quotations from the Grand Masters often contain archaic and or inconsistent use of language and syntax. My priority is to preserve their knowledge and wisdom, not to correct it. Therefore I have chosen in most of these instances to let their writings stand in their original composition.

Chapter 1
ANTIMONIUM TARTARICUM

Tartrate of Antimony and Potash

KEYNOTES

Mind Symptoms

- Extraordinary craving for apples and raw fruit (7)
- Child clings to those around (7)
- Child wants to be carried (7)
- Cries and whines if touched; will not let you feel the pulse (Antimonium crudum, Sanicula) (7)

Physical Symptoms

- Diarrhea after vaccinations (Silicea, Thuja occidentalis)
- Great accumulation of mucus in the air passages, with coarse rattling and inability to expectorate; impending paralysis of lungs (13)
- Great coma or sleepiness in most complaints (Opium, Nux moschata) (13)
- Thick eruptions: looks like pocks, often pustules; as large as a pea (13)
- Tongue is coated, pasty, thick, and white with red papillae and red edges; red in streaks; very red, dry in the middle (7)

- Child at birth pale, breathless, gasping for air; asphyxia neonatorium (7)
- Sound of "death-rattle" in a child (Tarantula) (7)

Aggravation

Worse: in damp, cold weather
Worse: cold
Worse: anger
Worse: morning
Worse: overeating
Worse: lying down at night
Worse: warmth in the room (Pulsatilla)
Worse: with the change of weather in spring (Kali sulfur, Natrum sulfur)

Amelioration

Better: cold open-air (Pulsatilla)
Better: sitting upright
Better: expectorating
Better: with motion
Better: after vomiting
Better: lying on the right side (Sulfur and Tabacum)

Causation

Effects of anger (cough) or vexation (10)

When Thuja Fails, and Silicea is Not Indicated

Dr. H.C. Allen clearly states that Antimonium tartaricum can be used for harmful vaccination effects when Thuja fails and Silicea is not indicated (7). Thuja is foremost in our minds regarding the destructive effects of vaccination. However, homeopathic doctors must think beyond Thuja, especially if the child is ill and has not made progress. Comparative Materia Medica is necessary to distinguish between remedies, as the selection may make a difference in the quality of life for the child.

Scars that Appear after Vaccination

The smallpox vaccination was launched and conducted by the World Health Organization from 1958 to 1977 to eradicate smallpox. One can still see the scar on an individual that has received a smallpox vaccination, as this scar is evident throughout life. We can learn from Dr. A. Pulford how he used homeopathic Antimonium tartaricum in succession to treat smallpox, followed by Thuja and Variolinum.

Antimony tartaricum or tartar emetic is very toxic, and when applied to the skin locally, it produces pustular eruptions. Dr. A. Pulford describes the pustular eruptions saying that it forms a scar identical to the scar that appears when receiving the smallpox vaccination. His description may be helpful when thinking of a remedy for a pustular eruption.

Dr. A. Pulford's notes have left detailed homeopathic writings that can help us select a remedy when the patient has received a vaccination that has left a scar on the individual. His notes are valuable for the treatment of smallpox and the history of the disease. According to Dr. A. Pulford, "The terrible backache of smallpox is paralleled in Ant-t. Ant-t. is said to correspond to more cases of lumbago than any other remedy. Crude Ant-t. rubbed into the skin forms a scar identical with that of vaccination. Ant-t. develops the smallpox, Thuja dries it up the smallpox, and Variolinum brings the whole affair to a speedy termination." (30)

Even though we don't see smallpox anymore, when working with Dr. Sarkar in his clinic in the village on the outskirts of Kolkata, I saw patients with a history of smallpox and the terrible scars it left on their faces and body. With the aftermath of smallpox and its symptoms, Dr. Sarkar was able to help the patients with a history of smallpox.

The Antimonium Tartaricum Child

The Antimonium Tartaricum Child is cranky and cannot tolerate anyone touching him. Like Chamomilla, the child wants to be carried by his mother and is quite clingy. With *The Antimonium Child* it is impossible to feel a pulse, listen to his lungs, or do a physical exam, as the child is troubled, agitated, and protests when approached.

This set of mind symptoms reminds me of Cina.

However, there is a difference. *The Cina Child* can be seen in my clinic, throwing himself on the floor, screaming, and flailing around. It is as if *The Cina Child* is having the worst temper tantrum of their life.

With Cina, worms, not vaccinations, are most likely at the source of this behavior. Remember, *The Cina Child* is a nose digger. The child is picking his nose because he or she may have a case of worms. Without a doubt, run an O & P (Ova and Parasite Stool Test) to confirm your suspicion. Cina is a gem with worms, the dreaded worms that cause such despair. What a blessing among remedies because Cina can battle an intolerable attitude, calm the worst temper tantrum, and eliminate those nasty worms.

Coughing Up Mucus

Perhaps this short keynote is the most outstanding. After a series of vaccinations, the child may develop large amounts of mucus in their airway. The mucus is stuck, rattling in nature, and the child cannot cough the mucus up. Here is the big clue. The parent tells you, "If my child could cough the mucus up, he clearly would be better." One may think of Sulfur first, but Antimonium tartaricum is the better choice. This keynote is the clue to healing and leads us to the selected remedy.

Newborn

The picture of the Antimonium tartaricum newborn or infant can be grave indeed. The newborn's description or picture is pale, breathless, and gasping for air. When alerted to these symptoms, think of Antimonium tartaricum as it may save the newborn's life. Dr. H. C. *Allen's Keynote* states, "Child at birth pale, breathless, gasping; asphyxia neonatorium. Relieves the 'death-rattle' (Tarantula)." (7)

Craving for Apples

One last note, *The Antimonium Tartaricum Child*, has an extraordinary craving for apples. This little gem has been helpful more than once. It gives the doctor confidence in the selection of medicine. Sometimes, the modalities provide us with confidence or lead the way. With that thought in mind, tell the parents to buy some Granny Smith apples for the child, and after treatment with Antimonium tartaricum, he might come around and show his sunny side.

Comparative Materia Medica

The following four remedies are essential to know and compare when treating the child that requires Antimonium tarticum.

Chamomilla

The child that requires Chamomilla is peevish and extremely irritable. He is quiet only when carried. The child is often labeled a child that is difficult to manage and extremely oversensitive. *The Chamomilla Child* can be oversensitive or temperamental from the use of medicines.

Keynotes to remember for Chamomilla:

- Peevish
- Extremely irritable
- Fretful
- Oversensitive
- Only quiet when being carried
- Impatient

Cina

The Cina Child is a cross and irritable child. Like Chamomilla, he wants to be carried. However, unlike Chamomilla, carrying does not comfort *The Cina Child.* Carrying does not bring relief. He does not want to be touched, and he rejects everything offered to him. You may see that *The Cina Child* regularly picks and digs in his nose.

Both Cina and Chamomilla have their place among the top remedies to prescribe when a child is hard to please.

Keynotes to remember for Cina:

- Cross and irritable
- Wants to be carried
- Carrying gives no relief

- Does not want to be touched
- Rejects everything
- Picks his nose

Silicea

Consider Silicea with harmful vaccination effects, especially when the patient presents with an abscess or convulsions. With Silicea there is a history of convulsions after the vaccination.

The child requiring Silicea is oversensitive. He is irritable, headstrong and obstinate. The child is chilly in temperature. The child has an offensive smell of the hands and feet. *The Silicea Child* desires to be magnetized (Phosphorus). Silicea is the chronic of Pulsatilla.

Keynotes to remember for Silicea:

- Oversensitive
- Irritability
- Head strong and obstinate
- Desires to be magnetized

Sulfur

Sulfur is a super remedy when thinking of the lungs. Sulfur helps facilitate the absorption of exudates in the brain, pleura, lungs, and joints. Sulfur is especially indicated when Bryonia alba, Kalium muriaticum, or the best-selected remedies fail. Sulfur is an essential remedy that must not be overlooked. Sulfur has deep healing actions.

The Sulfur Child cannot bear to be washed or bathed. All the child's symptoms are worse after a bath. Because Sulfur is a hot remedy one great keynote to remember is *The Sulfur Child* kicks off the bed cover at night. This keynote is similar to Hepar Sulfur and Sanicula. *The Sulfur Child's* feet are hot and you may see, to cool himself, he has put his feet out of bed while sleeping.

Sulfur is the grand collector. H.C. Allen states, "Everything looks pretty which the patient takes a fancy to; even rags seem beautiful. (7) *The Sulfur Child* is hungry at 11 a.m. (Zincum metallicum, Ignatia amara). They have an empty, all gone or faint sensation in their stomach and cannot wait to eat.

Consider Sulfur when selected remedies fail to produce the desired effect. Sulfur is the chronic of Aconite napellus.

Keynotes to remember for Sulfur:

- Cannot bear to be washed
- All symptoms are worse after bathing
- Kicks off the bedcovers
- A grand collector
- Hungry at 11 a.m.

Chapter 2
APIS MELLIFICA

Poison of the Honey Bee

KEYNOTES

Mind Symptoms

- Irritable, nervous, fidgety (7)
- Hard to please (Chamomilla, Cina) (7)
- Sudden, shrill, piercing screams in children while waking or sleeping (Helleborus) (7)

Physical Symptoms

- Vaccination site is swollen, sore, and stinging (7)
- Extreme sensitivity to touch (Belladonna, Lachesis) (7)
- Pain: burning, stinging, and sore in nature (7)
- All symptoms with no thirst (7)
- Puffiness of the affected part (7)

Aggravation

Worse: with bad news
Worse: touch or pressure, very sensitive
Worse: late in the afternoon
Worse: at 3 p.m.
Worse: heat of any form

Worse: after suppressed eruptions
Worse: after sleep (Lachesis)
Worse: in a closed, warm or heated room; child finds it intolerable (Pulsatilla)
Worse: from getting wet (Rhus toxicodendron)
Worse: on the right side
Worse: lying down

Amelioration

Better: washing or moistening the part with cold water
Better: open air
Better: cold water, cold application or cold bathing
Better: uncovering
Better: when sitting erect
Better: the head is better with pressure (this is an exception)

Causations

- Grief, fright, rage, vexation, and jealousy (10)
- Hearing bad news produces a mental shock (10)
- The queen bee is the most jealous thing in nature (10)

The Four S's: Sore, Swollen, Sensitive, and Stinging

Apis mellifica paints a clear physical picture after a child has received a vaccination or vaccination series. The injection area is sore, swollen, and is very sensitive to touch. If able to articulate their pain, the child will say that the area stings and burns. The pain with Apis is always sudden in onset and stinging in nature.

The child will feel better with a cool application on the swollen site, although they may refuse anything near the site of injection due to discomfort, sensitivity, and tenderness. Amelioration with a cold application differentiates Apis from Arsenicum album. Arsenicum is better with heat along with a hot application on the affected site. After vaccination, abscesses should put Apis at the head of one's list, providing the keynotes and modalities fit. If the child is better with a cold application, Apis can be considered.

One Busy Bee

The Apis Child, similar in nature to Cina and Chamomilla, is hard to please. *The Apis Child* is irritable, fidgety, and restless, and there may be plenty of tears after vaccination. The parent will describe the child as discouraged, upset, and sad.

The Apis Child colors a woeful picture indeed. "Getting a shot" from their doctor is bad news and can bring on fright and rage. We must not forget the mental image of Apis, as it is most disturbing. Apis has ailments from jealousy, fright, rage, vexation, and bad news. Who knows which comes first, the chicken or the egg, mental or physical symptoms? We must remember that Apis is the "Queen Bee." She gets easily upset and is very jealous.

As the progression of the illness occurs, you can see diarrhea, especially in eruptive diseases, and more so if the condition is suppressed. I shall not debate whether vaccinations are suppressive but rather leave this subject to the experts. They have more energy and indeed may prove to be wiser. Zincum metallicum can be considered in skin issues when there is a history of suppression from medicine or applied creams.

With homeopathic Apis mellifica and Comparative Materia Medica, the diarrhea is painless. This helps: rule out the painful diarrhea remedies first. Then select the medicine according to the time the diarrhea started: early morning diarrhea, diarrhea gets them out of bed, or a.m. and p.m. diarrhea. The selected remedy will be quite simple from there.

Questions Lead Us to the Right Remedy

- Is the diarrhea painful or not?
- What time did the diarrhea begin?
- Did the diarrhea begin in the a.m. or the p.m.?
- Did the diarrhea get them out of bed? (Sulfur)
- Is there urgency?
- Does the diarrhea episode occur after meals? (Thuja occidentalis)

Piercing Screams

Apis paints a more serious picture. We may hear piercing screams from the child as they sleep. The screams are very sudden and can be described as shrill, sharp, or high-pitched. The screams are disturbing. One must compare Apis with Helleborus as there is brain trouble in this example.

A high-pitched scream is often heard with autistic children. It is like none other, and perhaps it is the "crie cerebrale" that Dr. John Clarke describes in *A Dictionary of Practical Materia Medica*. The sound of their shrieks makes one think of brain inflammation, a profound disturbance that is often seen with a child requiring Zincum metallicum.

Dr. Clarke states, "Children constantly whining, screaming, sudden outcry during sleep. The stinging appears in many diseases and conditions, causing the "crie cerebrale" in acute hydrocephalus and meningitis." (10)

Dr. E. B. Nash gives us a clue, "The sleep of Apis is either very restless, or in brain disease there is deep stupor, interrupted occasionally by piercing screams."

Dr. E.B. Nash states, "In scarlatina, Apis is especially indicated if the eruption is retarded or retrocedent and serious brain troubles result, and it is no less efficacious in post-scarlatinal dropsies if the symptoms do not indicate some other remedies." (7)

Dr. Clarke states with Apis, "Hydrocephalus; scalp very sensitive; copious sweat of head; child lies in torpor, delirium interrupted by shrill cries, boring head deep in pillow, rolls it from side to side. Convulsed on one side of the body, paralyzed on the other." (10)

I worked with a Naturopathic doctor that gave Helleborus niger to every autistic child. Even I was surprised by the doctor's persistence, but the children all improved. Perhaps it is a lesson to learn. The power of Helleborus is important to remember and must be considered with one's differential diagnosis.

Apis Slow in Action

Apis is slow in action therefore confidence is needed with the selection of this remedy, especially when the child is so ill. Therefore, the remedy must be carefully studied by its keynotes. Stick with the remedy; don't switch. Have confidence. When the child starts to urinate or their pain decreases, you may let out a big sigh of relief, knowing that the remedy is working.

Apis: A Right-sided Remedy

Apis is a right-sided remedy. Apis has a progression that is right to the left (Lycopodium) and from above to downwards. The inoculation site will be worse if given on the right side.

The child will feel better in a cool room with a wet, cool application if permitted. Like Belladonna, the child will be worse at 3 p.m. The child often will feel better sitting up rather than on the couch watching television in a warm room with the window closed. Apis is similar to Pulsatilla in this respect. Both remedies are worse in warm, stuffy rooms.

Keynotes to remember for Apis:

- Apis is a right-sided remedy
- Right to left-sided progression
- Symptoms will appear from top to bottom
- *The Apis Child* will feel better in a cool room
- Wet, cool applications will help the affected area feel better
- Apis feels worse at 3 p.m.
- The child will feel better sitting up

Let the Modality Lead the Way

Let the modalities lead the way to the right remedy. When the homeopath is fortunate, the patient knows if he feels better with a cool or hot application. If not, ask them to try both hot and cold applications on the affected area. Patients are always surprised about such a little test. In most cases, the patient states the answer with great pride. That is the clue with Comparative Materia Medica. And that, My Dear Friend, makes a great homeopath even better.

Comparative Materia Medica

The following five remedies of Arsenicum album, Chamomilla, Cina, Pulsatilla, and Silicea are essential to know and compare when treating the child that requires Apis mellifica. The ability to understand the mind symptoms, physical symptoms, and modalities helps the homeopath in the selection of the remedy. Let like be cured by like.

Arsenicum Album

The Arsenicum Album patient presents with extreme physical weakness and emotional exhaustion. They tend to faint when ill or in a fearful state. They are extremely restless. The restlessness of Arsenicum is seen more often than any other remedy. Their anguish and severe suffering give them no rest. They can be observed going from place to place or bed to bed. This constant movement or restlessness further exhausts the patient. The patient has such anxiety that it drives him out of bed at night. The patient has a fear of death and thinks he shall die.

With an injury, vaccination, or acute disease, Arsenicum leads the way for burning pain. The burning pain is relieved by heat or a hot application. Arsenicum is a thirsty remedy and is better with cold water. Having stated this, the patient often drinks only small sips.

Keynotes to remember for Arsenicum Album:

- Great prostration and mental suffering
- Anxious, fearful
- Fear of death
- Restlessness
- Burning pain that is better with heat or a hot application
- Attack of anxiety will drive him out of bed at night

Chamomilla

The child that requires Chamomilla is peevish and extremely irritable. He is quiet only when carried. The child is often labeled a child that is difficult to manage and extremely oversensitive. *The Chamomilla Child* can be oversensitive or temperamental from the use of medicines.

Keynotes to remember for Chamomilla:

- Peevish
- Extremely irritable
- Fretful
- Oversensitive
- Only quiet when being carried
- Impatient

Cina

The Cina Child is a cross and irritable child. Like Chamomilla, he wants to be carried. However, unlike

Chamomilla, carrying does not comfort or bring relief to *The Cina Child.* He does not want to be touched, and he rejects everything offered to him. You may see that *The Cina Child* regularly picks and digs in his nose.

Both Cina and Chamomilla have their place among the top remedies to prescribe when a child is hard to please.

Keynotes to remember for Cina:

- Cross and irritable
- Wants to be carried
- Carrying gives no relief
- Does not want to be touched
- Rejects everything
- Picks his nose

Pulsatilla

Pulsatilla is a beautiful remedy for women and children. However, Pulsatilla is equally a man's remedy when the keynotes fit. The mental symptoms of Pulsatilla lead the way to the selection of the remedy. The patient is mild, gentle, and affectionate in nature. She is easily moved to laughter and tears. She weeps easily and is filled with emotions. Pulsatilla weeps as she narrates her story.

Pulsatilla has "ever-changing" symptoms. No two stools, menses, or chills are alike. Pain is ever-shifting and rapidly changing from one place to another. The more severe the pain, the colder the patient will be.

Pulsatilla is thirstless with all symptoms. The patient is worse with rich food, including cakes, pastries, sausage, and pork. The Pulsatilla patient is worse in a warm room. The Pulsatilla patient will feel better in a cool room, with a cool application. Eating cold food and drinking cold beverages will bring relief.

Pulsatilla is an excellent remedy to start a chronic case. Silicea is the chronic of Pulsatilla.

Keynotes to remember for Pulsatilla:

- Mild, gentle, and affectionate
- Impossible to detail her symptoms without weeping
- Quickly moved to laughter and tears
- Ever-changing symptoms
- Thirstless with all symptoms

Worse with fatty foods, pork, pasties and sausage

Silicea

Silicea may be helpful when there are harmful effects after a vaccination or vaccinations series. The patient can present with an abscess at the injection site or have a history of convulsions that began after a vaccination.

The child is oversensitive and will cry even when spoken to with a kind voice. The parent is likely to say their child is irritable, headstrong, and obstinate.

The Silicea Child is chilly. Their hands, feet, toes, and axilla sweat, and the smell is offensive. They have large heads and a history of open fontanelles and sutures. They are slow to walk.

The child will feel better when being magnetized, massaged, or stroked. They feel better when warm and their head is covered. Silicea is the chronic of Pulsatilla.

Keynotes to remember for Silicea:

- Silicea is mentally oversensitive
- Irritable, headstrong, and obstinate
- Child cries cry when spoken kindly to
- Silicea is chilly
- Offensive smell of the hands and feet
- Child desires to be magnetized or massaged (Phosphorus)
- A history of convulsions after vaccination
- Silicea is the chronic of Pulsatilla

Chapter 3
ARNICA MONTANA

Fallkraut, Leopard's Bane

KEYNOTES

Mind Symptoms

- Fearful of doctors (Ignatia amara, Natrum muriaticum, Stramonium, Thuja occidentalis)
- Patient says they are well when they are very sick (7)
- Nervous women, sanguine plethoric persons, lively expression, and very red face (7)
- Nervous, cannot bear the pain (Aconite napellus, Chamomilla, Coffea) (7)
- Great fear of someone approaching them (Belladonna, Stramonium, Thuja occidentalis) (8)
- Gout or rheumatism, with great fear of being touched or struck by someone coming near them (7)
- In children, they cannot have anyone come near them (Antimonium crudum, Cina, Cuprum)
- Aversion to being touched (Aconitum napellus) (8)
- Fear of crowds of public places; agoraphobia (Aconitum napellus)

- Aversion to answering questions (Hyoscyamus, Sulfur, Pulsatilla)
- Unconsciousness: when spoken to answers correctly, but unconsciousness and delirium after he answers (7) (8)
- Falls asleep amid a sentence (Baptista)
- Forgetful of words while speaking (Bothrops, Cannabis indica, Thuja occidentalis)
- Hunts for the correct words
- Indifference and apathy after concussion of the brain
- Memory loss after head injury
- Weak memory for what he has just said or what he is about to say.
- Mild personality
- Easily offended; takes everything personally (Calcarea, Carcinosinum, Lycopodium, Staphysagria, Tuberculinum)
- Refuses to take suggested medicine
- Oversensitive to external impressions, noise, and pain
- Children: shrieking, screaming, shouting during sleep (brain cry)
- Aversion to sympathy (the only remedy listed)
- Great sensitivity of the mind with anxiety and restlessness
- Whooping cough: the child cries before paroxysm of cough, fear of soreness

Physical Symptoms

- The whole body is sensitive (8)
- Cannot bear the pain (Chamomilla, Coffea, Ignatia amara) (8)
- Sore, lame, bruised feeling all through the body, as if beaten (7)
- Traumatic affections of muscles (7)
- Stupor from concussion; involuntary feces and urine (7)
- Concussions and contusions, results of shock or injury, without laceration of the soft part: prevents suppuration and septic conditions and promotes absorption (7)
- Compound fractures and their profuse suppuration (Calendula)
- Everything on which he lies seems too hard (7)
- Complains constantly of the hardness and keeps moving from place to place in search of a soft spot (the parts rested upon feel bruised and sore) (Baptista and Pyrogen) (7)
- Moves continually to obtain relief from the pain (Rhus toxicodendron) (7)
- Sensation of soreness of the arms
- Soreness of the whole body (10)
- Whooping cough: the child cries before the cough comes on (10)
- Affections of the brain
- Nose cold (10)
- Influenza (8)

- Arnica affects the left upper arm and the right chest (10)
- "Suddenness" is a feature of Arnica with pain and action
- Head and face hot, body and extremities cold (7)
- Stupor: answers then fall back into a stupor during a fever

Aggravation

Worse: damp, cold weather
Worse: least touch
Worse: motion and exertion
Worse: at rest
Worse: lying on the left side
Worse: with wine

Amelioration

Better: lying down
Better: lying down with the head low
Better: from contact

Causations

Injuries
Mechanical injuries
Fright or anger
Sexual indulgence
Vaccinations

Soreness after a Vaccination Series

After an injury, we can think of Arnica for first aid treatment. Arnica can also be considered after receiving a vaccination or a series of vaccinations. When Arnica is indicated, the injection site will feel bruised and swollen, leading the patient to extreme discomfort. The patient may state his arm is sore as if he has been beaten. *The Arnica Patient* may have an ecchymosis from the injection. When Arnica is given immediately after vaccination, the bruise may be avoided and the swelling minimal.

Going deeper yet, Arnica is indicated when the patient feels bruised all through the body after vaccination. He feels as if he has been beaten. Arnica may relieve the most persistent soreness and save the patient from further distress. According to Dr. H.C. Allen, Arnica is for the harmful effects of a mechanical injury, even if received years ago. The homeopathic doctor can think of a vaccination as a mechanical injury. Even if the injection site is painful or has a sensation of being bruised or beaten long after the initial injury, we must think of Arnica and its ability to heal.

Causation

The subject of causation in homeopathy is of utmost importance. Understanding the causation of an injury may lead straight to Arnica. A remedy can be prescribed on the causation alone, as with Arnica

Montana. According to George Vithoulkas, *Prescribing on Causation* is one of three ways of approaching or looking at a case.

George Vithoulkas states, "These causation symptoms can be considered very strongly. They are the starting points to finding the remedy, and a remedy must often be given that fits that causation even if it means ignoring other symptoms." (19)

Homeopathic Remedies Given on Causation

1. Arnica montana: conditions are resulting from injury (Bellis perennis, Conium maculatum, Lachesis)
2. Aconitum napellus: harmful effects from exposure to dry, cold weather
3. Dulcamara: illness resulting from hot days and cold nights
4. Hypericum: injury to nerves
5. Ignatia amara: ailments from grief
6. Natrum sulfur: ailments from anger, injury to the head, suppressed gonorrhea
7. Pulsatilla: bad effect from fatty food (Thuja occidentalis)
8. Staphysagria: bad effects from mortification
9. Thuja occidentalis: bad effects from vaccination

Bumps, Bruises and a Sore Sensation

Arnica is a crucial remedy for bumps that lead to a bruise or many bruises. Many keynotes have been listed so every possibility can be thought of when taking the patient's history and proceeding with a physical examination.

Dr. H.C. Allen states, "Weakness, weariness, sensation as of being bruised." (7) *The Sensation of Being Bruised* is a most critical keynote as there may not be a physical sign of the patient's bruise, but the patient states, "I feel bruised!" They tell you they feel sore and bruised or state that they feel sore all over their body, although the physician may not see signs of a bruise or a swelling.

Dr. E. B. Nash's Three Leading Pain Remedies (13)

- Aconite napellus
- Chamomilla
- Coffea

According to Dr. E. B. Nash, Aconite, Chamomilla, and Coffea are the three leading pain remedies. Here we must clarify that Arnica Montana is not listed as one of the three. However, Arnica is valuable in both acute and chronic diseases when there is pain. The keynotes lead the way for the selection of Arnica.

The Bed Feels Too Hard

The bed may feel too hard and leave the patient with an unusual sensation. *The Arnica Patient* is in pain with actual causation and a unique feeling. The discomfort causes extreme restlessness. The patient develops anxiety due to discomfort and pain.

Keynotes to remember for Arnica:

- The sensation of feeling bruised or sore all over, because the bed feels too hard, is real.
- Causes great restlessness as *The Arnica Patient* is in pain and cannot get comfortable.
- Because *The Arnica Patient* is so uncomfortable, they develop anxiety.

Treating Restlessness

When thinking of restlessness, we can look at Dr. E. B. Nash's writings. He clearly states and describes the three most restless remedies: Aconite napellus, Arsenicum album, and Rhus toxicodendron. His analysis is brilliant, and every homeopathic student can read it, as it will make the difference in selecting treatments. Arnica is not considered one of the three.

Dr. E.B. Nash also gives us additional information about this Trio of Restless Remedies, "All are so very equally restless, yet all are so very different that there is no difficulty in choosing between them."

Dr. E. B Nash's Three Leading Restless Remedies (13)

- Aconite napellus
- Arsenicum album
- Rhus toxicodendron

Arnica is not on the list even though *The Arnica Patient* is very restless. They cannot bear the pain

(Chamomilla, Coffea, Ignatia amara). Their pain, discomfort, and restlessness cause acute anxiety. This prompts the homeopath to compare Arnica with the leading anxiety remedies.

Aconite Napellus

When comparing Arnica, we can compare the remedy with Aconite napellus. The patient that requires Aconite is tossing about in agony and fear. They have a fear of death, crowds, and going out of the house. With Aconite, well, just about anything can cause a tremendous mental upset.

Aconite's anxiety begins with the onset or beginning of an illness or a fever. One more quote from Dr. H.C. Allen, one of our great masters of Homeopathy, "Aconite is a great pain remedy. The Aconite pains are always attended by extreme restlessness, anxiety, and fearfulness. The patient tosses about in agony."

Arsenicum Album

Arsenicum is the most restless patient found in the Materia Medica. As Dr. E. B. Nash states, "No remedy is more restless than this one." *The Arsenicum Patient* has extreme anxiety and is in complete anguish. Even if the patient is not in pain, he is so agitated that his mental state, of severe anxiety, drives him out of bed shortly after midnight. (12 a.m. to 2 a.m.)

Arsenicum has burning pain that is relieved by heat. It's such an unusual symptom which is why we must memorize this keynote. The pain that describes Arsenicum exhausts the patient. Instead of staying still, they move from place to place, from bed to bed. Their mental state is as great as their body pain.

Modalities are the most outstanding clue to look for when making a difficult decision. Arsenicum album is worse in the cold air, with a cold application, and most importantly, worse between 12 a.m. and 2 a.m.

If a patient wakes you with a phone call, just after midnight, in pain, have them apply a hot application to the area of discomfort. *The Arsenicum Patient* will describe the pain as burning in nature.

A hot application may not only calm the pain and reduce the patient's anxiety, but this little tip may give you more sleep. If the burning pain is worse from heat, dismiss the Arsenicum from your mind and move on. Suggest a cold application instead.

Influenza

In general, Arnica is a forgotten remedy during flu season. In America, nearly every household has the remedy tucked away with their medicinal supplies, in their knapsack, hiking equipment, or in their purse. Suffering could be diminished, with further instructions or confidence in the remedy's use. Patients think that

Arnica is just for injuries. They don't realize the in-depth actions of the homeopathic treatment.

As stated, Arnica can be considered after contracting influenza, receiving an influenza vaccination, or contracting a virus. The key or the secret with Arnica is understanding the most important keynotes. These keynotes help to solve the mystery of the remedy itself. Keynotes are essential when learning a remedy. They lead the way to the selection of Arnica versus another flu remedy that may not alleviate that particular patient's symptoms.

We must listen to each individual and note their symptoms as they may be quite different from another patient with influenza. We must keep in mind the differentiation or the comparison between other remedies.

Dr. H.C. Allen in *Allen's Keynotes* sums it all up in the first sentence in the Preface: First Edition. "The life-work of the student of the homeopathic Materia Medica is one of constant comparison and differentiation."

Comparative Materia Medica requires a lifetime of study and case taking that helps the doctor gain experience and confidence. The science of homeopathy is not for the dabbler, the weak-hearted, or the drifter.

Restlessness with Influenza

Another clue or keynote to consider that may lead the doctor to his prescription is restlessness in bed. *The Arnica Patient* cannot find a soft spot in their bed and feels as if the mattress is too hard. They feel as if there are lumps in their bed. This is the cause of his restlessness that, in turn, keeps him seeking the next comfortable spot.

However, Arnica does not have the restlessness of the remedy Arsenicum album. *The Arsenicum Patient* changes the bed, where *The Arnica Patient* changes the spot on or in the bed. *The Arsenicum Patient* wanders from place to place, where *The Arnica Patient* is just looking for that perfect spot, as the bed feels too hard, and they will say that their bed feels lumpy. *The Arnica Patient* stays in their bed, contrary to Arsenicum.

With Arnica, we must think of acute disease, bruises, and soreness sensations, but we must never forget chronic diseases or conditions where the patient has suffered for years. Arnica Montana is both for acute situations and a remedy for chronic conditions where the keynotes fit.

During an illness or influenza, a patient may keep changing his position. *The Arnica Patient* cannot get comfortable. Everything feels too hard against his body. The mattress feels too hard. The pillow is too hard; it brings distress. The patient is sure there are lumps in his bed.

Once again, there is nothing for the physician to see; the doctor must watch and listen to the patient. The doctor must observe the patient and think outside of the box.

When Arnica is indicated, the patient moves about, trying to find a better position to help the soreness. A doctor might think of Rhus toxicodendron in this example, but there is no stiffness, but rather the patient describes his discomfort as soreness as if having been beaten. Rhus toxicodendron is relieved with heat and stretching, but Arnica is not. Arnica is aggravated when resting, when lying down, in bed, and from wine.

Arnica, like Rhus toxicodendron and Ruta, is relieved by motion. Rhus toxicodendron has a rough beginning when moving, and the first few steps are difficult. Then the patient limbers up. *The Rhus toxicodendron Patient* is, in other words, lame and stiff. The pain is in the first motion; they feel better when moving more or gradually as they walk or get going.

However, *The Arnica Patient* is different as he cannot stay in bed. *The Arnica Patient* gets up to relieve the pain and the stiffness.

Keynotes to remember for Arnica:

- *The Arnica Patient* is uncomfortable
- The bed feels too hard
- The patient has a sore, lame, bruised feeling
- Feels as if they have been beaten
- Moving around to relieve the pain and stiffness

Comparing Arnica Montana with Ruta Graveolens

Ruta has a bruised, lame feeling all over. There is a history of injury or a fall and the lame, bruised sensation comes on after the incident. *The Ruta Patient* is uncomfortable lying down, and he feels bruised. They are restless and frequently change their position. Due to discomfort, they toss and turn which leads to agitation.

Ruta is an excellent remedy to complete the action of Arnica. If the bone has been affected or fractured, Ruta follows Symphytum nicely. Ruta heals the periosteum that covers the bone.

The Key to Arnica, Symphytum, and Ruta

- Give Arnica for the initial injury
- Symphytum for assistance to heal the fracture
- Symphytum is followed by Ruta
- Ruta aids the healing of the periosteum

When receiving an injection or a vaccination, if the needle is too long and the patient's arm is too thin, there may be an injury to the periosteum or the bone.

When the periosteum is damaged, Ruta may come in handy.

Ruta is a gem for dislocations. Ruta has an affinity for the wrist and the ankles. I have found out from experience if you choose Ruta, when Arnica would have helped, the patient will complain of throbbing that does not go away. At this moment, you must stop Ruta and select Arnica. With Arnica, the pain will completely go away. Above all, listen to the patient; they will tell you what heals, what makes them feel better, or what makes them feel worse.

Dr. C. M. Boger, written in Boger's: A Synoptic Key to Materia Medica, states in his keynotes for Ruta, "BRUISED, SORE, ACHING, and RESTLESS." (19)

Dr. Boger writes this in large caps to stress the importance!

- Ruta is worse from over-exertion, especially with a sprain or an injury
- Ruta is worse with the cold, damp, wet weather like Rhus toxicodendron
- Ruta and Rhus toxicodendron are both better with heat and a warm application

Allen's Keynotes says, "After Arnica, it (Ruta) hastens the curative process in the joints; after Symphytum in injuries to the bone." (7)

Comparing Arnica with Pyrogen

We can compare Pyrogen with Arnica when the keynote fits. "Everything that he lays on seems too hard." In this case, Pyrogen can be foremost in our minds during septic conditions where the patient is gravely ill. With Pyrogen, we will see the same symptom, the bed feels too hard, and the parts he lays on feel sore and bruised, like Arnica.

The Pyrogen Patient is extraordinarily restless and must continuously move to elevate the soreness. To distinguish the difference between the two remedies, one must remember that *The Pyrogen Patient* is gravely ill. This patient will have a very high fever and chills with septic symptoms and a rapid pulse. They are highly restless and can present with horrible, offensive discharges.

Introduced by English homeopaths, Pyrogen was prepared from decomposed lean beef and stood in the sun for two weeks. Then it was potentized. (8) Knowing the history of the remedy certainly helps the practitioner realize the depth of illness and, likewise, the healing nature of this remedy. Dr. H.C. Allen used this remedy and has left us with valuable keynotes. Dr. E. B. Nash states, "I have not used this remedy myself, but (if Allen's "Keynotes" are reliable) it must be of great value in affections of the most serious nature. A remedy recommended so highly, by such authority, for septicemia, puerperal, and surgical, and for diseases originating in ptomaine or sewer gas infection should not be passed lightly over."

Main points of Pyrogen

- Pyrogen is a nosode
- Pyrogen is a product of sepsis
- Pyrogen must be implemented with knowledge and care
- *The Pyrogen Patient* is gravely ill

Head Trauma

I will give a short history of a head injury case where Arnica was implemented with success. I had a young toddler of three in my clinic. She was diagnosed with autism. During the history, the parent had informed me the child had fallen out of her highchair at age two.

I started the case with Arnica. The mother argued with me, as many parents do. She was not happy with the selection of the remedy. She stated the child's fall was a year ago. She was sure I had selected the wrong prescription. I explain the keynote, "For the bad effects resulting from mechanical injuries, even if received years ago."

The parent still was not convinced. I explained we must treat *The Causation of the Disease first* then we can consider another remedy.

The little toddler received Arnica according to my directions. The following month, the family came back for their appointment. Was I ever surprised that the child greeted me by name as she skipped down the hall to my office. Her language had exploded. She had made astounding progress. Her sensory issues had decreased. For the first time, the child responded to her mother.

Under continued homeopathic care, the child progressed. At the last visit, her speech was appropriate for her age, and her vocabulary was vast. Her mother exclaimed that her child had bounding progress. The whole family was thrilled.

Note from Dr. M.L. Tyler

"A person who tires very easily and was knocked up by a day's shopping in London. Over fatigue always meant a bad night unless she took Arnica. On one occasion, she had been vaccinated, and her arm was swollen and sore, with painful glands in the armpit; on the top of which she had a dragging day in Town; so, at night, she took Arnica. To her surprise, she had no further discomfort from the vaccination! (Arnica is capable of producing cellulitis and septic conditions, and here it is relieved promptly.) Some of us always prescribe it, with relief to the patient, after a vaccination. Unlike Thuja, which aborts the process entirely, Arnica simply relieves the discomfort, leaving the pustules to take their usual course." (25)

Chapter 4
CARCINOSINUM

A Nosode from Carcinoma

KEYNOTES

Mind Symptoms

- Sleeplessness after vaccination
- A state of mental inactivity; lethargy (8)
- Mentally in an idle state: laziness and lassitude (8)
- Thinks with incredible difficulty (8)
- Indifference and apathy (Burnett)
- Experiences great fears (8)
- Sensitive to reprimands (Ignatia amara, Medorrhinum, Staphysagria) (8)
- Sympathetic to others (Phosphorus, Causticum) (8)
- Loves thunderstorms, cheerful and gay during storms (Burnett)
- Loves dancing (Burnett)
- Insominia or sleeplessness (Dr. Sarkar)
- Ailments from anticipation (Burnett)
- Fastidious (Burnett)
- Desires to travel (Burnett)

Physical Symptoms

- Never well since a vaccination or vaccination series
- Severe reaction to vaccinations
- Convulsions after a vaccination (Causticum, Cicuta virosa, Silicea, Thuja occidentalis, Variolinum)
- The child sleeps on their abdomen or elbows and knees (Medorrhinum) (Dr. Sarkar)

Aggravation

Worse: while undressing

Worse: cough from cold air, indoors

Worse: cough on the change from cold to warm or warm to cold

Worse: seaside air (Medorrhinum, Natrum muriaticum, Sepia)

Worse: ingesting honey

Worse: wet, windy weather

Worse: in a warm room

Amelioration

Better: rainy weather

Better: thunderstorms

Better: dancing

Better: seaside air

Better: in the evening

Better: stormy weather

Better: lying in knee elbow position

Better: with a short sleep

Causation

A history of an injury to the head (Foubister)
History of a concussion (Foubister)
Injury to the head at birth or during childhood
(Foubister)

History of Vaccination

Children in this day and age have a history of multiple vaccinations. When there is a history of vaccinations, this information can lead the prescriber to Carcinosinum. If the child has never been well after a vaccination series or has had a severe reaction to a particular vaccination, we can think about Carcinosinum.

Two important keynotes with Carcinosinum are sleeplessness after a vaccination or a history of convulsion with the vaccination. Causticum, Cicuta virosa, Silicea and Thuja must be considered when there is convulsion after a vaccination.

The child's mental state can also lead the prescriber to Carcinosinum. Here is an example. The child has difficulty learning. They are lethargic during their study period and indifferent to their subject. Parents may tell you that their child is lazy and does not have any incentive to learn or study. The child has a lack of motivation in general. Apathy is a great word that describes a child who can benefit from homeopathic Carcinosinum.

Dr. Sarkar states, "Children who need this remedy are precocious, mild, weeping, and gentle. They are a mixture of Ignatia and Lycopodium. We can also see the mind symptoms and gentleness of Pulsatilla."

Carcinosinum is a Nosode

Carcinosinum is a nosode from cancer pathology of the breast. Dr. W. Boericke lists Carcinosinum as "A nosode from Carcinoma." (8)

Dr. Sarkar gives the following application of a nosode which is considered when there is a strong history of infection:

1. The patient suffered from an infection, with no reaction after giving well-selected homeopathic medicines.
2. When the patient says, "I have not been well since an infection or illness."
3. When the same type of disease or infection repeatedly relapses, even after well-selected remedies or the constitutional remedy has been given.
4. During an acute infection, the nosode is given, along with an indicated remedy. This will cut short the disease process and prevent the disease's after-effects.
5. A nosode is prescribed on the homeopathic indication of symptoms, keynotes, modalities, and family history.
6. A nosode is considered when there is a pathological tendency with no clear indication.

Dr. Sarkar states, "Without the remedy Carcinosinum, it would be very difficult to heal cancer patients in today's generation. Most cases of cancer would need Carcinosinum 1M, 10M, and 50M, in ascending potentcies, even in acute conditions. This remedy is related to almost all polycrest remedies."

According to Dr. Sarkar, "A product of a nosode should not be the first prescription for the patient. First, one should implement the constitutional remedy and give the nosode as an inter-current. A homeopathic doctor prescribes the constitutional remedy first and then waits to see the results. 'Wait and Watch!' My students know this saying by heart. Don't be in such a hurry to prescribe the following medication. Let the remedy work. One must ask: Has the remedy produced favorable results? Does the patient feel better?"

Dr. Sarkar also teaches, "Follow the first remedy or the constitutional medicine with the nosode. There must be a time in between the two treatments. Carcinosinum is a potent remedy."

Dr. Sarkar continues, "After prescribing Carcinosinum, give the remedy time. That means time for the remedy Carcinosinum to do its work. There must be time for healing. Do not hastily hurry to another remedy. Being hasty with your prescription is not the answer."

Rules for prescribing Carcinosinum in review:

- Give the patient a constitutional remedy first
- Give time for the remedy to work

- Give Carcinosinum as an inter-current
- Let Carcinosinum work and give time for the body and mind to heal

A Physical Picture

According to Dr. Sarkar, "The child may not have any major history of an illness during childhood. There is no history of measles, mumps, chicken pox or any of the childhood diseases usually seen in the early years of the child's life. This is an important observation as it can be part of a pattern of confirmatory keynotes that I use to prescribe Carcinosinum."

The Carcinosinum Child may have multiple birthmarks. Birthmarks are common in a child that will make progress on Carcinosinum. Observing a keloid formation, Port-wine stains, or a child with numerous moles can lead to the remedy Carcinosinum. In other words, observation gives us the first clue but does not stop there.

According to Dr. Sarkar, "All skin symptoms are worse undressing. The skin symptoms the child has will be worse at the seaside. We must keep in mind that the Carcinosinum patient may have recurrent abscesses, a history of fistulas, sinus infections and keloids.

Physical signs to consider:

- Keloids: easy scarring
- Many moles
- Birthmarks
- Port-wine stains

Swinging Symptoms

The Carcinosinum Child can have swinging symptoms. What does this mean? There are many physical and mental symptoms, but the symptoms are never consistent; they constantly change. For instance, there can be a swing in the child's temperature preference. Sometimes the child feels hot, and sometimes the child feels cold. One minute the child feels hot and rips his jacket off, and five minutes later, he cries because he feels cold. He wants socks and a blanket. He wants to cuddle.

Swinging symptoms are observed with a child's appetite. Sometimes the child is hungry, and sometimes he is not. When the child is not hungry, he will flat-out refuse to eat. I have given this scenario a name. I refer to this as *hungry days and not hungry days*. Parents understand this concept and catch on to the name quickly as they have seen this scenario with their children many times.

With swinging symptoms, suddenly, there is a reverse. The child's symptoms can go in the opposite direction—what a surprise. For the homeopathic doctor, this information, lack of information or confusing information makes it challenging to understand which way the case is going. Difficulties arise during the case taking when swinging symptoms appear. There is no head or tail, no beginning or end to the case. Swing symptoms lead the case taker to confusion. Confidence shrinks. The doctor may doubt his credibility when taking a case that requires Carcinosinum.

We see swinging symptoms with two other remedies, Pulsatilla and Berberis. A comparison is necessary between these remedies. It is up to the homeopath to decide.

Swinging symptoms according to Dr. Sarkar:

- Temperature variations (the patient is chilly and then too hot)
- Hungry to no hunger
- There is a totally opposite direction of symptoms
- Symptoms are on one side of the body and then switch to other side
- Constipation to diarrhea and vice versa
- No two stools are the same
- One minute happy, the next minute the patient has mind symptoms of a tropical storm

A Mental Picture

Mentally, Carcinosinum is a most exciting remedy.

I shall paint a picture of one of our most prominent nosodes. *The Carcinosinum Child* is fearful. The child suffers greatly. Their fear persists despite play therapy and other interventions. Although the child's fears torture him, at the same time, the child loves thunderstorms. Amazing! Why, you ask? It is because thunderstorms are loud, sudden, and unpredictable. Thunderstorms are dramatic. They can scare the bravest adult.

The Carcinosinum Child is cheerful and gay, happy and excited, filled with delight when there is thundering and lightning. A child that is fearful but loves thunderstorms is contradictory. Dr. Sarkar explains, "The Carcinosinum patient enjoys rainy weather. It would not be unusual to find the child dancing in the rain."

Emotional Trauma and Grief

There is often emotional trauma with deep-seated grief behind *The Carcinosinum Child's* symptoms. With contradictory signs, Ignatia amara comes to mind. Ignatia is the remedy of great contradictions. Both Ignatia and Carcinosinum share the symptom of long, concentrated grief.

Shared symptoms of Ignatia and Carcinosinum:

- A history of emotional trauma
- Deep-seated grief

- Long concentrated grief
- Contradictory symptoms

The Carcinosinum Child may have difficulty thinking, concentrating, comprehending, and doing well in school. They get easily confused. They are dull, sluggish, and have great problems thinking. The child thinks with incredible difficulty.

They can be labeled as the "Discontented child." *The Carcinosinum Child* is easily displeased and cannot tolerate any contradiction.

- *The Carcinosinum Child* is intolerant of contradiction.
- The child is easily offended and takes everything with a negative attitude (Burnett).
- *The Carcinosinum Child* is very sensitive to reprimanding.

Everyone around them, including parents, relatives, doctors, therapists, and teachers, notices the child's obstinate, headstrong behavior. "My way or the highway!" behavior is difficult for everyone. The worst part of this scenario is that the child is worse and easily aggravated with consolation.

Remedies for children sensitive to reprimands:

- Ignatia amara
- Medorrhinum

- Staphysagria
- Natrum muriaticum

One can consider Staphysagria with an easily offended child, but Carcinosinum may bring more in-depth results. Comparative Materia Medica steps to the forefront with these two remedies, Staphysagria and Carcinosinum. The homeopathic doctor has many decisions to make.

When the Case Leaves the Doctor Puzzled

When taking a child's case, there are symptoms, keynotes, and indications for the remedy Carcinosinum. Here is the clue. When sitting and observing the child and considering all of the parents' input, the doctor becomes PUZZLED. It appears that this child has three constitutional remedies. For example, Zincum metallicum, Sulfur, and Calcarea carbonica seem equally indicated. There is also a family history of cancer. Bingo! A family history of cancer is an indication to apply the nosode Carcinosinum.

Another scenario popped up during my case taking when I was a younger doctor. However, it was not a frequent happening. I ask you, what is the worst thing that can happen to a homeopath taking a case? There is *No Lead to a Remedy*.

I took the child's case meticulously, but there was no particular remedy leading the way to the prescription.

Tracing the keynotes to a specific medication was difficult. What was I going to do? Oh help, I would think silently under my breath. My throat got tight from anxiety. However, to complete the patient's full history, a homeopath must take the full family history. Ah, I still had the family history left to take. After listening and recording the family history, I discovered a family history of cancer. The puzzle started to unravel. Suddenly the case made sense. I had great confidence and was able to apply my prescription.

My office manager taught me a saying, "The show is not over until the fat lady sings!" In other words, case-taking is not over until the family history is complete. Every detail is essential. The family history can undoubtedly link to the application of a nosode.

Dr. John Clarke had a fascinating opinion; he stated that Carcinosinum is more indicated than any other nosode. Dr. William Boericke goes on to explain, "It is claimed that Carcinosinum acts favorably and modifies all cases in which either a history of carcinosinum can be elicited, or symptoms of the disease itself exist (J. H. Clarke, MD). Dr. Sarkar states, "You can give Carcinosinum when there are multiple miasms present. For example, the patient may have a history of cancer, tuberculosis, malaria or diabetes."

Chapter 5

HEPAR SULPHURIS CALCAREUM

Hahnemann's Calcium Sulphide

KEYNOTES

Mind Symptoms

- Excessive irritability (7)
- Oversensitive, physically and mentally (7)
- The slightest cause irritates him (7)
- Quick, hasty speech and hasty drinking (7)
- Great sensitivity to all sense impressions (8)
- Peevish, angry at the least trifle (7)
- Hypochondriacal, unreasonably anxious (7)

Physical Symptoms

- Suppuration at the slightest injury (Graphites, Mercurius) (7)
- Skin is very sensitive to touch (7)
- Cannot even bear clothes to touch his affected parts (Lachesis is sensitive to the slightest touch) (7)
- Skin affections extremely sensitive to touch; the pain often causes fainting
- Craving for sour and strong-tasting food in children

- Diarrhea with sour smell (Calcarea, Magnesia carbonica) (7)
- Child and stool have a sour smell (Rheum palmatum) (7)
- Clay-colored stool (Calcarea, Podophyllum) (7)
- Sweats profusely day and night
- Itching, upper limbs, after abuse of mercury
- Rheumatic pain after abuse of mercury

Aggravation

Worse: lying on the painful side (Kali carbonicum, Iodum)
Worse: cold, dry winds
Worse: cold air and slightest draft
Worse: in dry weather or the least little wind
Worse: uncovering in general and uncovering the head
Worse: on single parts of the body getting cold
Worse: eating or drinking cold things
Worse: touching affected parts
Worse: from any form of mercury
Worse: nighttime
Worse: during sleep
Worse: on awakening
Worse: blowing the nose
Worse: from surgical injuries in general
Worse: from getting the skin rubbed off
Worse: from daylight
Worse: application of mercury

Amelioration

Better: warmth in general (Arsenicum album)
Better: wrapping up the body warmly
Better: wrapping up the head (Psorinum, Silicea)
Better: warm air
Better: in damp, wet weather (Causticum, Nux vomica, the reverse of Natrum sulfur)
Better: after eating

Causation

- Cold, dry wind
- Injuries
- Mercury in all forms: dental amalgam, medicines, or preservatives used in vaccinations
- Suppressed eruptions

Periodicity

- Every day
- Every four weeks (attack of paralysis)
- Every four months (scabies eruption on the head)
- Spring and autumn (bilious attacks)
- Every winter (whitlows)

Over-Sensitive is the Grand Picture

Over-sensitive is the grand picture of Hepar Sulfur. *The Hepar Sulfur Child* is sensitive in body, mind, and soul. The inoculation site is very sensitive to the slightest touch. Furthermore, the child cannot bear any clothing touching the vaccination site. The skin is difficult to heal, and it is extremely sensitive.

Dr. H.C. *Allen's Keynotes* states, "The slightest injury causes suppuration (Graphites and Mercurius)." With each vaccination, the sites flare up and cause much distress for the child and those around him. The reaction is immediate.

The true definition of flare-up is a sudden outburst of symptoms. We must not forget, with Hepar Sulfur, the explosion is in both body and mind. Hepar Sulfur has the flame and intensity of symptoms no one will forget. Due to *The Hepar Sulfur Child's* exaggerated response, everyone around the child will quickly become aware of his physical and emotional pain. Due to their over-sensitive manner and extreme physical symptoms, the child is like a desert dust storm. You can see it coming, but you cannot get out of its way fast enough.

Not only is the child sensitive to touch but the slightest draft of air is unbearable. *The Hepar Sulfur Child* is also highly sensitive to noise and odors. This is a perfect picture of *The Highly Sensitive Child*. The child is touchy in body and mind. The child is upset. He is the *unhappy camper* with himself and anyone around. Irritable, angry, and emotionally touchy are the descriptors that fit this child's mood.

The Hepar Sulfur Wet Barking Cough

I often prescribe Hepar Sulfur for a wet barking cough. Hepar Sulfur is a gem of a remedy and nothing short of a miracle in my practice. This particular cough is aggravated by a cold morning and the marine layer of the San Francisco Bay Area. The smallest breath of the cold morning air brings on what I call *The Hepar Sulfur Wet Barking Cough.*

Dr. Clarke states, "Hepar croup is accompanied by a rather loose cough, wheezing and rattling. Cough as if mucus would come up, but it does not. The time of the Hepar croup is early morning (Aconite in the evening). The least breath of cold air worsens the cough or any uncovering."

We never know how deep a homeopathic remedy works, but I dare say that Hepar Sulfur works VERY DEEP. The application of Hepar Sulfur is essential with children that have been diagnosed with autism. For proper application, the indications and keynotes must be present. With Hepar Sulfur, the change is in both the body and mind. While treating *The Hepar Sulfur Wet Barking Cough*, we treat a foul mood, extreme sensory issues, and the accumulation of mercury that is present in the body. That, my friend, is a VERY DEEP medicine indeed.

Mercury: Notes from the Great Masters

The great masters of homeopathy have left us with useful information, keynotes, and observations on Hepar Sulfur and its application for mercury toxicity. Hepar Sulfur has a long history of treating mercury toxicity or the symptoms of mercury toxicity. Mercury is a neurotoxin. Children exposed to methylmercury in utero may develop devastating effects on their cognitive thinking, memory, attention, language development, fine and gross motor skills and visual spatial skills.

Uses of Hepar Sulfur

- Dr. H.C. Allen states, "Diseases where the system has been injured by the abuse of mercury." (7)
- Dr. H. C. Allen writes, "Hepar antidotes: bad effects of mercury and other metals; iodine, iodine of potash, cod-liver oil." (7)
- Dr. Clarke states, "Its antidotes: Metals, especially mercurial preparations, Nitric Acid, Calcarea, Iodum, Kali iodum, Cod-liver-oil." (10)
- Dr. Clarke tells us, "In this connection, it may be well to speak of the relation of Hepar to Mercurius. Hahnemann's instinct led him to see in Hepar an antidote to mercurial poisoning, and it remains still the chief antidote, whether to the effects of massive doses or over-action of the potencies." (10)

- Dr. Clarke states, "In 1794, Hahnemann proposed to use it (Hepar sulfur) internally to arrest mercurial salvation." (10)
- Dr. Clarke states, "Antidotes for Hepar Sulfur: metals, and especially mercurial preparations." (10)

Strange, Rare, and Peculiar Symptoms

Strange, rare, and peculiar symptoms help the homeopath select a remedy. Time and time again, Dr. Sarkar tells his student how valuable these symptoms can be. For instance, on a hot, humid afternoon in Dr. Sarkar's Salt Lake Clinic, a young patient in his 20's came in with extreme pain. There were so many sick patients in the clinic and numerous emergencies ahead of this young man. He was lying on the ground, on the floor in the clinic. He was in extreme pain. He was so chilly he was shaking and crying out in pain.

Dr. Sarkar asked me to attend to the patient until he was free. Do a physical and take his history. The patient did not speak English. Things were difficult for me to understand. Dr. Sarkar called me back into his room and asked me what was wrong with the patient and what remedy could I suggest. I was not sure.

Finally, Dr. Sarkar was free. He noticed that with increased pain, the patient became chillier. With a short intake, the patient received his prescription: Pulsatilla. The patient recovered in a short period. Dr.

Sarkar said to me, "The patient had increased chilliness with his pain. Could you not see that?" It was apparent to Dr. Sarkar, and as for me, I had a lot to learn. Dr. Sarkar saw many patients per day, and many times his clinic was more like a homeopathic Emergency Room. One had to think quickly.

I leave you with a few strange, rare, and peculiar symptoms as they may come in handy in the future. They sure have for me.

Summary of strange, rare, and peculiar symptoms to remember:

- Pulsatilla: with increased pain, there is increased chilliness
- Chamomilla: with increased pain, there is increased sweating
- Hepar Sulfur: with increased pain, there is fainting
- Veratrum Album: with increased delirium, there is increased pain

Chapter 6
MAGNESIUM PHOSPHORICA

Phosphate of Magnesia

KEYNOTES

Mind Symptoms

- Children: exhausted, tired, and have difficulty thinking clearly
- Aches after mental labor, patient is chilly afterwards (8)
- Inability to think clearly (8)
- Sleeplessness due to indigestion (8)

Physical Symptoms

- Ailments after Tetanus vaccination (14)
- Lockjaw (10)
- Prevents lockjaw (Hypericum) (8)
- Cramping muscles and radiating pain (8)
- Spasms during dentition: no fever (7)
- Tetanic spasms (8)
- Convulsions (10)
- Stiff and numb in arms, hands, and fingertips (8)
- Muscular weakness (8)
- Affections on the right side of the body (Belladonna, Lycopodium, Apis mellifica) (7)

- Pains are sharp, cutting, stabbing, shooting, and stitching (Belladonna) (7)
- Pains come on like lightning: come and go quickly (7)
- Colic: flatulence, the child bends double, better with heat, rubbing, and hard pressure (7)
- Cramps: of extremities, during pregnancy, with writing, playing the piano, or violin (7)

Aggravation

- Worse: on the right side
- Worse: cold, cold air, cold winds, and cold weather
- Worse: cold bathing or washing
- Worse: lack of clothing
- Worse: touch
- Worse: standing in cold water
- Worse: after working with cold clay (Calcarea Carbonica)
- Worse: light touch of the affected part
- Worse: headache: worse lying down
- Worse: studying
- Worse: uncovering (Hepar Sulfur, Rhus toxicodendron)
- Worse: movement
- Worse: night
- Worse: dentition

Amelioration

- Better: with heat and warmth
- Better: warm or hot application (Silicea, Arsenicum album)
- Better: bending over double (Colocynthis)
- Better: pressure
- Better: friction
- Better: hot drinks

Causation

- Dentition
- Cold winds
- Cold bathing
- Standing in cold water
- Working with cold clay
- Studying too long
- A history of catheterization

The Use of Magnesium Phosphorous after Vaccination

Magnesium phosphorus may bring relief after inoculation with the tetanus vaccination. After receiving a vaccination, there may be spasms or contractions of the fingers. These spasms will be predominately on the right side of the body. This is because Magnesium is predominantly a right-sided remedy that is its most predominant modality. Cramping pain is characteristic of this remedy but should be compared to Cuprum and Colocynthis.

- An excellent anti-spasmodic remedy (8)
- Pain relieved by warmth, warm application (7)
- The remedy acts exceptionally well in hot water
- The headache is always better with a warm application
- Better with cold application contraindicates Magnesium phosphorus

Headaches after Vaccination

For the treatment of headaches, let me quote Dr. H.C. *Allen's Keynotes*, "Headache that begins on occiput and extends overhead (Sanguinaria canadensis, Silicea); of schoolgirls; face red, flushed, from mental emotion, exertion or hard study; worse 10 to 11 a.m. or 4 to 5 p.m.; better by pressure and external heat." (7)

The key for prescribing Magnesium phosphorus may be in its modalities. For example, a right-sided headache that started after a vaccination may lead us to Magnesium phosphorus. The vaccination is the causation, and the headache is better with a warm application.

Modalities introduced by Dr. Clemens Von Boennninghausen, MD give the homeopath important information and help with selecting the remedy. Whether the symptom is ameliorated or aggravated may lead the doctor right to the remedy. Magnesium phosphorus is a right-sided remedy that is better with warmth and a warm application. Modalities in this case and with many remedies are of the utmost importance. Headaches can be diverse in pain, giving the homeopath a real challenge. Knowing the remedy modalities may lead the way and provide confidence in a prescription.

Dr. John Clarke states the description of Magnesium phosphorus and its application in a way the homeopath is not likely to forget. "Headache: pains shooting, darting, stabbing, shifting; intermittent and paroxysmal. Headaches: excruciating; spasmodic; neuralgic or rheumatic; always better by external application of warmth." (10)

The two main points of Dr. Clarke's description:

1. The headache can vary with symptoms, diversity, and intensity.
2. The modality leads the way to the correct prescription.

Dr. Clarke's descriptions of the diverse symptoms of a Magnesium Phosphorus Headache (10)

- Headache better towards evening: changes to pressure above the eyebrows, especially on the right side
- Headache beginning in or worse in occiput, and constant while attending school
- Severe headache: face flushed red; pain began in occiput, extending over the whole head; sick at stomach; aches all over; worse 9 to 10 a.m. to 4 or 8 p.m.
- Pressing headache down through the middle of the brain
- Pain through the temples, top, and back of the head, with a sensation of fullness, worse lying down
- Sensation of a strong shock of electricity beginning in the head and extending to all parts of the body
- Severe headache began in occiput on waking, extending over the head, located over both eyes, with severe nausea, and terminated at 5 p.m. in a pronounced chill

Diverse Pains

Pains of Magnesium phosphorus can be diverse; therefore, let us not be confused. Dr. E.B. Nash describes diversity well. "Magnesia phosphorus takes the first rank among our very best neuralgia or pain remedies. None has a greater variety of pains. They are sharp, cutting, piercing, stabbing, knife-life, shooting, stitching, lightning-like in coming and going (Belladonna), intermittent, the paroxysms becoming almost intolerable, often rapidly changing place and cramping." (13)

- Sharp and shooting pain
- Darting pain
- Stabbing pain
- Shifting pain
- Intermittent pain
- Paroxysmal pain
- Excruciating pain
- Spasmodic pain
- Neuralgic pain
- Throbbing on the vertex
- Pain deep within the brain
- Dull headache: as if the brain were too heavy
- Pain: rheumatic in nature
- Nervous headache

Headache for the Doctor

I have decided to bone up and read all I can on Magnesium phosphorus. Every homeopath would be wise to do the same. As Dr. Sarkar has reminded me more than once, "Headaches are a headache for the doctor."

My answer to Dr. Sarkar is always the same, "Please don't say that, as you know, I get terrible headaches."

I must say in the same breath, as soon as my headache begins, I reach for Magnesium phosphorus, and it seems to make the difference. Again, the remedy selection is pointed out in the modalities. My headaches are ever-changing, stabbing, shooting, and every other description known to man. They are worse with touch, massage, and lying down. I follow the remedy with a nice cup of hot tea and pretend I am with the Queen of England. That seems to make a difference and puts me in better spirits.

Fatigue and Exhaustion

Fatigue is a common symptom associated with Magnesium phosphorus. As Dr. Sarkar tells me, "You will find with Magnesium phosphorus that the patient is dog tired. They are so tired they can hardly sit up. Think of a doctor such as myself; the patients are lined up at the door, my fingers have cramps from writing notes and by the hundredth patient, I no doubt am fatigued and feel like lying down. It is a sense of exhaustion beyond belief. Perhaps I should take a dose of Magnesium Phosphorus myself."

Dr. H.C. Allen quotes in *Allen's Keynotes*, "Languid, tired, exhausted; unable to sit up." (7)

Dr. John Clarke states under Generalities, "Convulsions: whooping cough; spasms without fever; crampy contractions of fingers; staring, open eyes. Every twenty-three days, spasms. Tired easily; shooting, tingling, electric pains all over the body. The student is asleep or drowsy when studying. They have an inability to think clearly and are very forgetful." (10)

The Modality Leads to the Remedy

Of utmost importance, Magnesium phosphorus's modality can be a leading character with any pain or discomfort. Magnesium phosphorus is relieved with warm, heat, or hot application. If the patient is relieved with a cold application, then Magnesium phosphorus is contraindicated and the presumed remedy must be immediately dismissed.

A Perfect Picture of Magnesium Phosphorus

When describing a perfect picture of Magnesium phosphorus after a set of vaccinations, such as the DTaP (diphtheria, tetanus, and pertussis), think of the patient with spasms or cramps. The muscle cramps may radiate or travel, causing extreme discomfort. The right side of the body may be affected, and the patient will have increased discomfort with the cold wind or cold application. They are relieved with warmth, heat, and hot application.

We must thank Dr. Clemens Von Boenninghausen, MD for his diligent work in formulating the principle that the cure is in the modality. For example, one application of a modality might be: Have the patient sip on hot water after taking Magnesium phosphorus.

Sipping hot water may make a difference and bring relief to the patient.

Comparative Materia Medica

Cuprum Metallicum

Cuprum displays spasms and cramps that appear and disappear in groups. These cramps are located in the extremities, soles of the foot and calves and produce great exhaustion. Tonic and clonic spasms begin in the fingers and the toes and spread all over the body. These cramps can be seen in pregnancy and puerperal convulsions. The causation is fright, anger, rage, or vexation. There can be cramps in the patient's hand.

Symptoms start on the left side of the body. Magnesium phosphorus symptoms begin on the right side and proceed to the body's left side. This progression is similar to like Lycopodium.

The modalities are different than Magnesium phosphorus, as Cuprum is worse before menses and from vomiting. Cuprum is better during perspiration and drinking cold water. Magnesium phosphorus is better with heat, hot water, and drinking hot drinks.

The opening note stated by Dr. Boericke, in the *New Manual of Homoeopathic Materia Medica & Repertory*: "Spasmodic affections, cramps, convulsions, beginning in the fingers and toes, violent, contractive and intermitting pain, are some of the more marked expressions of the action of Cuprum, its curative range, therefore, includes tonic and clonic spasms, convulsions and epileptic attacks." (8)

Keynotes to remember for Cuprum metallicum:

- Spasm and cramps: symptoms disposed to appear periodically and in groups
- Cramps in the extremities: pains in the soles of the feet, calves with great weariness
- Convulsions with a blue face and clenched fist
- After pains: severe distress in calves and soles of the feet

We can differentiate remedies that have twitching or jerking of a single muscle, or remedies that appear to have spasms in groups of muscles. Cuprum, may I repeat, displays spasms and cramps that appear and disappear in groups. Other remedies that must be compared with Cuprum include Zincum metallicum, Agaricus muscarius, and Ignatia amara. These three remedies apply to twitching and jerking of a single muscle. This may help with a differential diagnosis. One more note that is important, copper is found in plants such as Solanum Dulcamara or Bittersweet, Delphinium Staphysagria, and Conium maculatum which is our Poison Hemlock.

Colocynthis

The Colocynthis Child has shooting pains like lightning.

The pain goes down the whole limb, left hip, left thigh, knee, and into the popliteal space. Again, just a reminder that Magnesium phosphorus is a right-sided remedy. The right side goes to the left like Lycopodium, but I have already written this, so please be tolerant, not like Colocynthis. At times we see the clue of the remedy in the modalities.

Agonizing pain in the abdomen causes the patient to bend over double. *The Colocynthis Child* is better with hard pressure, whereas Magnesium phosphorus is better with heat. Colocynthis is an irritable child that throws things. They are incredibly impatient and are angry or quickly offended if questioned.

Keynotes to remember for Colocynthis:

- External impressions: light, noise, strong odors, contact, bad manners, make him almost beside himself (Nux vomica)
- The child's suffering seems intolerable
- Ailments: from grief or misdeeds of others (Staphysagria, Lycopodium)
- *The Colocynthis Child* may have sensory issues that can easily upset them
- Sensory issues can include light, loud noises, strong odors, and touch
- The child angers quickly
- Like Staphysagria, Colocynthis has ailments from grief and indignation

Chapter 7
MALANDRINUM

A Nosode: The Grease of Horses

KEYNOTES

Mind Symptoms

- Confusion and lassitude of the mental faculties
- Dread of any mental exertion and a lack of concentration
- Comprehension difficult
- Memory weakened and impaired
- Great difficulty in remembering what was read
- Melancholy with general fatigue
- Sensation of weariness at the junction of the atlas with cranium; every morning on rising

Physical Symptoms

- Pustular eruption on the scalp
- Itching on the scalp, especially in the evening
- Excessively oily dandruff
- Impetigo covering the head from crown to the neck and extending behind the ears

- Thick greenish crust with pale, reddish scabs, that itches in the evening
- Impetigo that covers the back of the head, extending over the back to the buttocks, labial, and into the vagina

Aggravation

Worse: in the evening (Dr. R. Straube)

Causation

Vaccination (Dr. Straube)

Malandrinum: The Forgotten Remedy

Dr. John Clarke leaves us with one word under causations. "Vaccination." (10) He has put this statement in singular form, as the smallpox vaccine was the first vaccination and the only vaccination at the time this remedy was proven and then written. Hopefully, my writing and thoughts will give the reader something to contemplate. I certainly had to work my little gray cells; now it is your turn.

I have to admit, I have thought about the remedy Malandrinum for months upon months before taking up my pen to write. A question that made me ponder was whether or not to include Malandrinum in this book because of its complexity and infrequent application. Frankly, the remedy Malandrinum fascinates me. The keynotes may make a difference when trying to understand this remedy and its complexity of symptoms.

Malandrinum is such a necessary remedy. Dr. Sarkar states all in the same breath, "Malandrinum is a forgotten remedy, little used. Malandrinum stands in the pharmacy with other nosodes that are rarely used."

What is Horse Grease?

Malandrinum or *Grease of the Horse* is a nosode. Dr. John Clarke tells us that the nosode comes directly from the disease or the lesions on the horses. He referred to this disease as *Grease*.

Grease of the Horse is known today as Mud Fever. Mud Fever is dermatitis that develops in the lower limbs of horses. Many bacteria can cause *Grease* or Mud Fever, including Dermatophilus congolensis and Staphylococcus. *Grease of the Horse* or Mud Fever can also be caused by a fungal organism. Other names for *Grease of the Horse* include dew poisoning, grease heel, or greasy heel. (32)

The appearance of *Grease* seen in horses is described as red, inflamed, and oozing in nature. If left untreated, the skin can become infected and sore, causing the lesion to crack and deepen. Horses are more likely to contract Mud Fever or Grease in the winter and spring when they stand in ponds or muddy water. Their skin becomes compromised. The lesions grow and develop scaling with a crusty formation, hair loss, edema, and oozing. (32)

Introduction of Malandrinum

Dr. H. C. Allen writes, "Dr. Boskowitz, of Brooklyn, was the first to introduce and use Malandrinum. He made the first potencies up to the 30th from the crusts of the *Grease of the Horse*. To the observations of Dr. Boskowitz in the use of this remedy, both as a prophylactic and therapeutic remedy against smallpox and the bad effects of vaccination are added those of

Dr. Raue, Carleton, Smith, Wm. Jefferson Guernsey, Selfridge, Wesselhoeft, Burnett, and Clarke." (7)

According to Dr. H.C. Allen, "The remedy has had extensive proving by W. P. Wesselhoeft, H. C. Allen, Steere, Holcombe, and students of Hering College, in 1900 and 1901." (7)

The homeopathic remedy, Malandrinum, can be considered with ill vaccination effects. In general, the application of Malandrinum is useful when the keynotes fit, in a case presenting with acne, boils, fistulas, impetigo, measles, and other skin issues. When we see signs of a Staphylococcus infection, we can think of the remedy Malandrinum. Signs of Staphylococcus infection include redness, swelling, itchiness, and tenderness at the lesion site. If advanced, lesions can present with pus, oozing, or crust covering the open site.

Upon studying Malandrinum, we can see that it has an affinity for the mind, head (headaches), ears, nose and throat, gastrointestinal system, and skin. Malandrinum has leading keynotes that can help the ill effects of vaccination, and therefore we must once again bring the remedy into view and consideration.

When considering the modalities, we must consider Dr. Rudolph Straube's proving. He noted that all symptoms are worse in the evening. Dr. Straube did his proving with the 30th potency.

With this short introduction, let us look at the keynotes. Keynotes are short little snips of information that leave us thinking. They help us with the selection of a remedy and guide us to the simillimum.

For Bad Effects of Vaccination: (5)

- For ill effects of vaccination, this remedy has been used with the best results (8)
- When used as a prophylactic for variola has proved protective in many cases, and has prevented vaccination from "taking"
- Has cured cases of unhealthy, dry, rough skin, remaining for years after vaccination in smallpox, measles and impetigo (10)

Difficulty Learning

This set of symptoms left by the provers and the great masters of homeopathy made me sit up straight and wake up. We will see that the child requiring Malandrinum has trouble learning. The patient is confused and tired. *The Malandrinum Child* dreads any mental work and has a definite lack of concentration. The child has difficulty concentrating, and comprehension is difficult. Their memory is weak and impaired. *The Malandrinum Child* has great difficultly remembering what they have read. They dread any mental exertion at all.

Keynotes to remember for Malandrinum:

- Confusion and lassitude of the mental facilities
- A dread of any mental exertion and a lack of concentration
- Difficulty during an entirely new and unusual experience that continues several weeks after stopping the remedy
- Comprehension is difficult
- Memory is weak and impaired
- Great difficulty in remembering what was read
- Lack of concentration
- Dread of any mental exertion
- Melancholy with general fatigue
- Sensation of weariness at the junction of the atlas with cranium; every morning on rising

Ill Effects of Vaccination

Clarke states, "It has been used on inferential grounds with great success in ill effects of vaccination (I have cured with it, cases of unhealthy, dry, rough, skin remaining for years after vaccination)." (10) Dr. Clarke used the nosode specifically in smallpox, measles, and impetigo.

Dr. William Boericke gives us two comparisons with his keynote: Ill effects of vaccination (Thuja occidentalis, Silicea). Short but sweet, he adds, "Malandrinum is very effective in preventing smallpox." (8)

Dr. Clarke gives us a little history, "According to Jenner, the origin of cow-pox is an infection of the udders of cows by contact with grass on which a horse infected with *Grease* has trodden. This assertion is to some extent confirmed by the experience of homeopaths, who have found in Malandrinum very effectual protection against infection with smallpox and against vaccination." (10)

Dr. H. C. Allen in *Materia Medica of The Nosodes with X-Ray Provings* adds more history. "Jenner noted that it was from the unwashed hands of the stable "neys" who milked the cows after grooming the horses infected with Grease. These assertions are to some extent confirmed by the clinical experience of many homeopaths, who have successfully used Malandrinum against infection with smallpox, and for the bad effects of vaccination." (25)

Once again, Dr. H. C. Allen confirms with his keynote, "For the bad effects of vaccination has been used with best results." (25)

One interesting piece of history from Dr. H. C. Allen, "Malandrinum was given to 600 persons, many of whom had been exposed by personal contact with various patients, before and after taking the medicine; only one case of so-called varioloid (smallpox) occurred, and this may have been a proving of Malandrinum." (25)

In his provings, Dr. Straube lists under Skin: Bad effects of vaccination. We are not left with any details, but according to Sherman, Tex, February 20th, 1900, "It may be well to begin with the paper in 1883, as it contains the result of the provings arranged in an orderly manner. In a few introductory words, Dr. Straube warns the reader not to think that Malandrinum is derived from "Malanders" in the horse, as some have; it is simply the "grease" virus of the horse potentized according to the rules of homeopathic pharmacy." Malanders or Mallenders is an old-fashioned term for cracks in the skin behind the horse's knee.

Cancer Treatment

Once again, as with other remedies, we have a hint. Dr. Robert Thomas Cooper, a well-known Irish physician of his time (1844-1903), leaves us with a short keynote to ponder, "Efficacious in clearing of the remnants of cancerous deposits."

Dr. Cooper was an intense lover of plants. He potentized plants, then developed, and applied the remedies clinically. He used the remedies he potentized to treat cases of cancer. He was known to take on complex cases and had great success in his clinical practice.

We are left to wonder about the rest of this note and how Malandrinum will aid the patient with cancer. In this case, one must consider the remedy as a whole with all of its keynotes. The key may be in the patient's history. The history of vaccination for smallpox may be the beginning or the causation of the disease. One last note, in the original provings by Dr. Rudolf Straub, under Skin records: smallpox, measles, also preventive. He adds in: malignant pustule. It is with this short note, containing no details, that Dr Cooper may have begun his work.

Malandrinum can be considered with bone cancer where there is boney protuberances or exocytosis. But of course, Hekla Lava must be on the forefront when there is a boney protuberance, protrusion, or exocytosis. I have already written about Hekla Lava in *Monsoon Medicine: Keynotes & Materia Medica.*

Comparative Materia Medica

When there are ill effects of vaccinations, other remedies should be compared, such as Vaccininum, Variolinum, Thuja occidentalis, Sabina, Antimonium tartaricum, Apis mellifica, and Silicea.

With symptoms of severe sore throat, Malandrinum can be compared with Belladonna. Dr. Straube explains that Stramonium can be considered when there are keynotes and indications such as hallucinations and delirium in severe smallpox cases.

Cases written by Dr. R. Straube describe what it was like to treat patients using Malandrinum. He treated many highly complicated cases of smallpox. His provings were extensive and carried out on 20 healthy patients. His provings were done with the 30th potency.

Dr. R. Straube writes in his proving of Malandrinum, "Follows well with Bryonia, Lachesis, and Stramonium. After Malandrinum, Silicea is often indicated (perhaps Tartar emetic)."

Chapter 8
SULFUR

Brimstone, Flower of Sulfur

KEYNOTES

Mind Symptoms

- Children: cannot bear to be washed or bathed (7)
- Restless
- Everything looks pretty, which the patient takes a fancy to (7)
- Rags seem beautiful (7)
- Children who collect everything
- Kicks off the clothing at night (Hepar sulfur, Sanicula) (7)
- Happy dreams, wakes up singing (7)

Physical Symptoms

- Eruptions following vaccinations
- Children: prone to skin affections (Psorinum)
- Child has worms: consider when the best-selected remedies fail to work (7)
- Constant heat on vertex (7)
- Cold feet in the daytime with burning soles at night, wants to find a cool place for them (Sanguinaria canadensis, Sanicula)

- Puts their feet out of bed to cool them off at night (Medorrhinum)
- Diarrhea: drives the child out of bed early in the morning (Aloe, Psorinum) (7)
- Constipation: stool is hard and knotty, dry as if burnt (Bryonia alba)
- Stool: large and painful (7)
- Child afraid to have the stool on account of pain (7)
- Stool: pain compels the child to desist on the first effort (7)
- Child has alternating constipation and diarrhea
- Parts around the anus red and excoriated
- All the orifices of the body are very red (7)
- Skin voluptuous itching, better scratching, but the scratching causes burning (7)
- Skin: itching worse with the heat of the bed (Mercurius) (7)

Aggravation

Worse: at rest
Worse: when standing
Worse: in the warmth of the bed
Worse: washing or bathing
Worse: bathing in the morning
Worse: at 11 a.m.
Worse: at night
Worse: periodically
Worse: from the abuse of metals
Worse: scratching

Worse: touch, pressure

Worse: after drinking milk

Worse: with changing weather (Rhus toxicodendron)

Worse: cold, damp weather

Worse: talking, that causes fatigue of the whole body

Amelioration

Better: lying on the right side (reverse of Stannum metallicum)

Better: from drawing up the affected leg (Thuja occidentalis)

Better: dry skin

Better: motion

Better: doors and windows open (Pulsatilla)

Better: dry, warm weather

Causation

- Suppression
- Alcohol
- Sun
- Sprains
- Chills
- Over-exertion
- Reaching high
- Falls
- Blows
- Bedsores

Relationships

- Sulfur is complementary with Aloe and Psorinum
- Sulfur is compatible with Calcarea carbonica, Lycopodium, Pulsatilla, Sarsaparilla, and Sepia
- Calcarea must not be given before Sulfur
- According to Dr. S. Sarkar, Sulfur, Calcarea, and Lycopodium are to be given in this order
- Aconitum napellus is the acute of Sulfur
- Sulfur frequently serves to rouse the reactive powers when carefully selected remedies fail to act (especially in acute diseases, in chronic, Psorinum) (10)

Introduction

When a child is diagnosed with autism, Asperger's syndrome, or ADHD, homeopathic Sulfur is one of the most incredible remedies our Materia Medica has to offer. I have listed many keynotes for Sulfur. Each keynote is important, leading the homeopath to the remedy that decreases the suffering of a child on the spectrum. Each keynote can lead to the simillimum.

We, as homeopaths, must realize that Sulfur is at the top of the list for the child that has had harmful effects from a vaccination or vaccination series. Consider the power of Sulfur. Sulfur can be implemented as a constitutional remedy, an acute remedy for present symptoms, or as a prophylactic. Sulfur can be used as a preventive remedy to protect the child from a vaccination's harmful effects (Thuja occidentalis, Variolinum).

Sulfur has produced remarkable results when prescribed for children. The remedy has helped children with developmental delays, learning, tantrums, speech, and reading. Sulfur heals in the physical body and the mental plane. In my practice, the benefits, or miracles, of Sulfur as a homeopathic remedy have been endless.

Sulfur: A Cornerstone of Homeopathy

Dr. Sarkar reminds me that Sulfur, historically, was once referred to as *the fire of Sulfur* and is one of three cornerstones of our homeopathic Materia Medica.

Sulfur, Calcarea carbonica, and Lycopodium make up this triangle's trio.

Dr. Sarkar repeats a phrase to memorize, "Sulfur-Calcarea-Lycopodium. *S-C-L*, for short, is a gem to remember the relationship of this cornerstone. Don't be too proud to say this trio to yourself before prescribing. I say *S-C-L* often. Saying *S-C-L* reminds me of the order of prescription. Over the years, saying *S-C-L* has worked for me. With this advice, the patient will heal in fashion according to Hering's Law of Cure."

The Law of the Directions of the Symptoms

Dr. Constantine Hering, the father of American Homeopathy, taught us *The Law of the Direction of Symptoms*. *The Law of the Directions of the Symptoms* is essential to remember:

- From an organ of more importance to a less important one
- From within outwards
- In the reverse order of the symptoms appearing
- From above downwards

Not only must the parent of a child learn that the healing order is essential, but many doctors must be reminded. The most important organs are the brain, the heart, and the lungs. I will include the intestines here. Eighty percent of the immune system is located in the intestines. These organs must heal first.

The Law of the Directions of Symptoms tells us the patient must heal from within outwards. The Law states that the organs such as the brain, the heart, or other deeper organs must heal before the skin. The brain must show signs of improvement before a skin rash has healed. Symptoms of brain healing include improved speech, comprehension, and decreased irritability.

The last part of *The Law of the Directions of Symptoms* states that healing must take place from above downwards. A rash heals from top of *the head to bottom. The Bottom* can be interpreted as the hands, fingers, and feet or toes. Extremities or digits will be the last part of the body to heal.

Case Example

I shall tell you of a beautiful case that is an example of *The Law of the Directions of Symptoms*. During medical school, we gave a patient homeopathic Lachesis. The prescription was given for a bad case of eczema. All principles were followed. We asked the patient to return one month later for a follow-up visit.

The patient's healing followed *The Law of the Directions of Symptoms* to the letter. Dr. Sarkar thought this patient's healing was a fundamental lesson. He asked all the students in the clinic to come, see, and learn. "*Just you see!*" he explained to the patient and the students, "Her direction of healing, from above downwards, is a beautiful example of *The Law of the Directions of Symptoms*." Dr. Sarkar was very pleased indeed: the eczema receded from her waist and moved down to her toes as she was healed.

I see *The Law of the Directions of Symptoms* with patients many times per month. I get so excited for the child and the parents. I have to explain my excitement, and the beauty of their child's healing as the parents wish for eczema to heal first and have trouble understanding that learning, comprehension, and speech must lead the way and are more critical.

After prescribing homeopathy, especially homeopathic Sulfur, I see children progress. The child learns, develops increased muscle tone, and catches up with their milestones. Often, the speech therapist tells me they are beginning to speak or have made extensive progress. This all happens before their eczema is healed. According to *The Law of the Directions of Symptoms*, this is the right order outlined and taught by Dr. Hering.

I explain Hering's *Law of the Directions of Symptoms*, to parents during return visits. The parents hold on to every word. They learn fast. *The Law of Cure* is essential. Explanations give the parents hope, encouragement, and patience. If the lesson is skipped, the parents expect the skin to heal first.

Use of Sulfur for Vaccination Symptoms

Dr. Clarke states, "In the early days of vaccination, it was found that the action of Sulfur on the frame was decidedly averse to the receptivity of vaccine. According to Dr. Tierney, Dr. Jenner failed in vaccinating thirty soldiers, all under treatment by Sulfur. (B.M.F., Jan. 6, 1872. George Gascoin, letter on the antiseptic treatment of smallpox)." (10)

Dr. James Kent states, "The dreadful effects of vaccination are often cured by Sulfur. In this it competes with Thuja and Malandrinum." (12)

Hypersensitive Skin

Sulfur has an affinity for the skin. This remedy alleviates many skin symptoms such as:

- Burning
- Itching
- Worse with any heat: whether there is an application of heat or from the heat of the bed

After vaccination, the skin appears red. Like Hepar Sulfur, any injury or vaccination suppurates and becomes troublesome. There is swelling and extreme discomfort after immunization. The inoculation site is over-sensitive, and the child will complain.

According to Dr. Clarke, "Another manifestation of this is found in the redness of orifices and parts near orifices: red ears, red nose; red eyelids and red borders around eyelids: brilliant red lips; bright red anus in children; red meatus urinarinus; red vulva." (10)

Redness is the key. Itchy skin. The child feels better scratching the area but soon regrets the action as immediately the site burns and becomes much worse. Dr. E. B. Nash states in his keynotes, "Skin: Itching, voluptuous; scratching; > "feels good to scratch"; scratching causes burning; < from the heat of bed (Mercurius)." (13)

Sulfur is well selected when the prescriber is challenged, and other remedies have not improved the patient's health. The remedy acts in acute and chronic diseases and can clear the case. We can think of Sulfur when symptoms continually relapse. When the patient is doing well and then has a turn for the worse we can think of homeopathic Sulfur. When properly selected, Sulfur helps a child with developmental delays and assists a child in reaching their milestones.

Guiding Skin Symptoms

- Eruptions on the skin after a vaccination
- Congestion in the affected area
- Sensations of burning, heat in and around the vaccinated area
- Vaccinated area is worse with any heat or hot application
- All skin symptoms worse after scratching

- Worse from the heat of the bed or when the covers become warm
- Worse when bathing or washing the vaccination or affected area

Aversion to Taking a Bath or Washing

Sulfur Skin is best left alone as everything irritates the skin. For instance, the skin is worse washing or bathing, worse washing with medicated soaps, and worse scratching. A parent will soon find out the child has hypersensitive skin. The wound, vaccination site, or area that the child has scratched is better left alone.

Sulfur is indicated when suppressed eruptions cause the disease or discomfort. We have one reminder from Dr. E.B. Nash's keynotes, "Dirty, filthy people, prone to skin affections (Psorinum)." (13)

After the child has received a vaccination, the doctor can hang a sign around the child's neck, "Do not touch, scratch, or bathe me. I am better left alone! Please, do not be tempted."

Dr. Clarke makes one statement that has stood up against time, "Children who cannot bear to be washed or bathed." All trouble starts from here. (10) Should I dare say that with a bath, all trouble breaks loose? A keynote reminds me, "Skin: symptoms of burning that lead to scratching lead to more burning." It is a hopeless situation, which is only to be relieved by homeopathic Sulfur.

Comparative Materia Medica

There is a trio of burning remedies that must be considered in our comparison Materia Medica. *Arsenicum album, Phosphorus, and Sulfur* lead the way. It would be best if you distinguished between these. I will leave you with a few clues.

Arsenicum Album

Arsenicum album is our top burning remedy. Dr. E. B. Nash puts the burning remedies in a classification that include Arsenicum, Sulfur, Phosphorus, Acid sulfur, Cantharis, and Capsicum.

The Arsenicum Album patient presents with extreme physical weakness and emotional exhaustion. They tend to faint when ill or in a fearful state. They are extremely restless. The restlessness of Arsenicum is seen more often than any other remedy. Their anguish and severe suffering give them no rest. They can be observed going from place to place or bed to bed. This constant movement or restlessness further exhausts the patient. The patient has such anxiety that it drives him out of bed at night. The patient has a fear of death and thinks he shall die.

With an injury, vaccination, or acute disease, Arsenicum leads the way for burning pain. The burning pain is relieved by heat or a hot application. Arsenicum is a thirsty remedy and is better with cold water. Having stated this, the patient often drinks but in small sips.

Keynotes to remember for Arsenicum Album:

- Great prostration and mental suffering
- Anxious, fearful
- Fear of death
- Restlessness
- Burning pain that is better with heat or a hot application (the opposite of Sulfur)
- Attack of anxiety will drive him out of bed at night

Phosphorus

Phosphorus can present with a weak, empty, all-gone sensation in the head, chest, stomach, and entire abdomen. Their burning spots are all along the spine and between the scapulae. The patient may state that they have intense heat running up the back and on the palms of the hands. Phosphorus is better with cold drinks and cold food. Juice is refreshing and ice cream helps with gastric symptoms.

The Phosphorus patient feels better in the dark, lying on the right side. They feel better when rubbed or mesmerized.

Keynotes to remember for Phosphorus:

- Burning sensations are worse on the left side
- Worse when touching the affected site
- Worse lying on the left or painful side
- Better washing with cold or cold applications (the opposite of Sulfur)

Chapter 9
THUJA OCCIDENTALIS

Arbor Vitae: Tincture of the fresh green twigs

KEYNOTES

Mind Symptoms

- Absent-minded, forgetful
- Answers questions slowly
- Angry, irritable, and quarrelsome
- Angry when contradicted
- Filled with anxiety
- Fixed ideas: as if a strange person were at his side, aversion to touch (7)
- Aversion to company
- Avoids the sight of people
- Aversion to the presence of strangers
- Concentration is difficult
- Confusion of the mind
- Confusion of the mind in the morning
- Dullness of the mind
- Difficulty with the thought process
- Makes mistakes in writing
- Emotionally sensitive (8)
- Craves company (8)
- Music causes weeping and trembling

- Illusion of shape (Baptisia tinctoria, Petroleum, Stramonium)
- Aversion to touch or approach (a fixed idea) (Antimonium tartaricum)

Physical Symptoms

- Eruptions only on the areas with clothing (7)
- Diarrhea: early morning, worse after breakfast (7)
- Diarrhea: after eating potatoes, onions, or fatty food (rich food: Pulsatilla)
- Diarrhea: after vaccinations (Antimonium tartaricum, Silicea) (7)
- Diarrhea: expelled forcibly with a lot of flatus (Aloe socotrina, Natrum sulfuricum)
- Chronic otitis media: purulent discharge (7)
- Chronic runny nose: catarrh: thick and green (7)
- Asthma in children
- Very sensitive to touch
- White scaly dandruff
- Hair: dry and falling out
- Nails soft (Fluoric acid)
- Persistent insomnia
- Ophthalmia neonatorum (neonatal conjunctivitis)

Aggravation

Worse: in the afternoon
Worse: at night, after midnight
Worse: early morning (the sycotic time)

Worse: at 3 a.m. and 3 p.m. (worse at 3 p.m.: Apis mellifica, Belladonna)
Worse: with or during damp weather
Worse: from cold, wet, and damp weather
Worse: on becoming cold, on exposure to cold air
Worse: after breakfast, after eating
Worse: from tea, coffee, and beer
Worse: sweets
Worse: from onions, pork, rich, and fatty food or fatty meat
Worse: from the smell of food
Worse: during rest
Worse: from narcotics or tobacco
Worse: from or after vaccinations
Worse: from the moonlight and the moon increasing
Worse: sunrays, sunstroke, or becoming overheated
Worse: bright light
Worse: from the heat of the bed (Apis mellifica, Mercury, Pulsatilla, Sulfur)
Worse: touch (Scalp, vertex, eruptions, anus, condyloma acuminatum)
Worse: blowing the nose (pain inside of the teeth)
Worse: jarring, stepping
Worse: use of Sulfur
Worse: extension of the limbs
Worse: gonorrhea, badly treated or suppressed
Worse: sexual excess

Amelioration

Better: lying on the left side
Better: while drawing up a limb (Sulfur)
Better: moving
Better: with touch
Better: with heat, warm and dry
Better: in the open air
Better: headaches are better from rest

Causation

- Vaccination
- Gonorrhea badly treated or suppressed
- Sunstroke
- Sexual excess
- Tea
- Coffee
- Beer
- Sweets
- Tobacco
- Fat meat
- Onions
- Sulfur
- Mercury

Relationship with Other Remedies

Complementary: Arsenicum album, Medorrhinum, Natrum Sulfur, Sabina, Silicea

Compare with other Hydrogenoid Constitutional Remedies:

Aranea diadema, Apis mellifica, Calcarea carbonica, Natrum Sulfur, Pulsatilla, and Silicea

Chronic of Silicea: Thuja occidentalis

Introduction

Thuja occidentalis is one of our most essential homeopathic medicines. After years of studying Thuja, I realize it is crucial to share the most important keynotes and application of this remedy. Thuja has an amazing healing potential and cannot be substituted with other remedies. Therefore, with all sincerity, let us begin to unravel the mysteries of Thuja and its application regarding the bad effect of vaccination or a vaccination series.

I have used Thuja occidentalis extensively in my practice. I am not sure where life, medicine, and homeopathy would be without this remedy. In the state of California, the law requires vaccinations. I support and implement preventive treatment as needed.

Thuja occidentalis is the *Tree of Life* which treats many problems that begin with vaccination's destructive effects. Common symptoms such as diarrhea, constipation, or skin rashes can appear after a vaccination or a vaccination combination. Perhaps a child has never been well since a particular scheduled vaccination series. For example, if anxiety, depression, or other mental symptoms developed after a vaccination, Thuja can be implemented. Thuja will help with symptoms that started after the vaccination.

Thuja occidentalis: Bad Effects from Vaccination

Thuja occidentalis has left-sided symptoms with a few exceptions. There can be right-sided atrophy of the arm after vaccination, oozing from the right ear, smelling like putrid meat, swelling of the right side of the tongue, and affection of the right abdominal ring.

It is important to remember that Thuja is a strong left-sided remedy. The patients usually have one-sided complaints, such as paralysis on the left side. Children are most likely vaccinated on the left arm, which increases the chance of having swelling and tenderness on the left arm. The question is whether or not Thuja is a left-sided remedy because most children are vaccinated on the left side. This is an issue to ponder and for experts in the field to debate.

Uses of Thuja to remember:

- From bad effects or ill effects of vaccinations (Antimonium tartaricum, Apis mellifica, Carcinosinum, Pyrogen, Silicea, Sulfur, Vaccininum, Zincum metallicum) (7)
- Never well since vaccination (13)
- Abuse of mercury (Aurum metallicum, Carbo vegetabilis, Hepar sulfur, Kalium iodatum, Lachesis, Natrum sulfuricum, Phytolacca decandra, Staphysagria, Sulfur, Zincum metallicum)

The Doctrine of Causation

Homeopathy places great importance on causation. Dr. C. M. Boger introduced *The Doctrine of Causation* into homeopathy. According to Dr. Boger, "Correct prescribing is the art of carefully fitting pathogenetic to clinical symptoms, and as such at present requires a special aptness in grasping the essential points of symptom images, great drudgery in mastering a working knowledge of our large Materia Medica or a most skillful use of many books of reference." (19)

Following Dr. Boger's model, homeopathic Thuja can be implemented or introduced as a causation remedy. According to Dr. Boger, one can address *"The Causation of the Disease"* or symptom first. (19)

Dr. Boger writes, "The spirit of the clinical symptom picture is best obtained by asking the patient to tell his own story, whenever this is possible. This account is then amplifying and more accurately defined by the question, who should first try to elicit the evident cause and course of the sickness, to which he will add all the things which now seem to interfere with the sufferer's comfort." (19)

Dr. Boger's Modalities include:

- Causation
- Time
- Temperature

- Weather
- Open air
- Posture
- Motion
- Eating and drinking
- Sleep
- If alone
- Pressure
- Touch
- Discharges

In *Lectures on Homoeopathic Materia Medica,* James Tyler Kent states, "Thuja is pre-eminently a strong medicine when you have a trace of animal poisoning in the history, as snake bite, small-pox, and vaccination." (21)

Dr. Sarkar states, "Anytime there is a new protein, even a blood transfusion, introduced into the body, we must think of Thuja occidentalis as an antidote. Thuja may be the antidote and go on to save the patient's life."

For progress with the patient, *one must address The Causation of the Disease. The Causation of the Disease* is a vital principle of homeopathy. Thuja occidentalis will strengthen the vital force and restore the patient's health.

Dr. Clarke states under Thuja: Causation of Disease, "Vaccination. Gonorrhea badly treated or suppressed:

sunstroke, sexual excess, tea, coffee, beer, sweets, tobacco, fat meat, onions, sulfur, mercury." (10)

In the *New Manual of Homoeopathic Materia Medica & Repertory* by Dr. William Boericke listed under Modalities, the list includes: "Worse at night, from the heat of bed: at 3 a.m. and 3 p.m., from cold, damp air, after breakfast; fat, coffee; vaccination." (8)

Dr. Boericke lists a straightforward word in his introduction: the last line, under Thuja, "Vaccinosis, viz., inveterable (chronic, long-standing) skin problems, neuralgia." (8)

George Vithoulkas explains there are many different methods of prescribing or looking at a case: (20)

- By looking at the essence. This is the main idea of the case, the theme that runs through all the symptoms.
- By looking at the totality of the symptoms.
- By looking at the keynotes. These are the peculiar and unusual symptoms.
- By looking at the causation, e.g., if a patient tells me that her skin eruption started after her child died or his stomach problems started after losing his job, then this is the CAUSATION.

George Vithoulkas states, "These causation symptoms can be considered very strongly. They are the starting points to finding the remedy, and a remedy must often be given that fits that causation even if it means ignoring other symptoms."

Once again, Dr. Sarkar reminds the homeopath to sit up and pay attention, "Thuja can be prescribed as an inter-current. For instance, perhaps a child has had eczema ever since a particular vaccination. This child can be given Thuja followed by the specific remedy for the child's eczema or perhaps his or her constitution remedy."

Homeopathic Remedies Given on Causation

Arnica montana: Conditions resulting from injury (Bellis perennis, Conium maculatum, Lachesis)

Aconitum napellus: bad effects from exposure to dry, cold weather

Dulcamara: illness resulting from hot days and cold nights

Hypericum: injury to nerves

Ignatia amara: ailments from grief

Natrum sulfur: ailments from anger, injury to the head, suppressed gonorrhea

Pulsatilla: bad effect from fatty food (Thuja occidentalis)

Staphysagria: bad effects from mortification

Some remedies, but not all, in homeopathy can be prescribed on causation. The science of homeopathy gives great importance to causation. Thuja occidentalis is an example of a remedy that can be prescribed on causation. When the causation of a problem or a disease is from the harmful effect of vaccination, Thuja can be implemented. If a parent describes the child's illness and, in the same breath, describes the onset of symptoms after giving a vaccination, then Thuja can be implemented.

Chapter 10
THYROIDINUM

Sarcode from the Thyroid of a Sheep or Calf

KEYNOTES

Mind Symptoms

- Depression (7)
- Despair of recovery (7)
- Slow thinking
- Stupor, alternating with restlessness and melancholy
- Irritation with the least little opposition (8)
- Goes into a rage: over slightest little trifle (8)
- Difficulty with memory
- Indifference to everything (Sepia, Phosphoricum acidum)
- Euphoria alternating with quarrelling
- Desire to lay down: does not wish to do anything
- Fretfulness and moroseness: giving way to cheerfulness and animation (7)
- Ill-tempered (7)
- Angry (7)
- Fearful
- History of a fright (7)

- Malaise better by lying in bed (7)
- Insomnia (7)

Physical Symptoms

- Cold hands and feet (8)
- Dry, cracked, brittle nails
- Desires sweets (8)
- Weight gain
- Constipation (10)
- Hair loss, thinning hair
- Swelling of the face and legs (7)
- Angioedema (8)
- Edema of the legs (7)
- Goiter (7)
- Hypothyroidism after acute illness
- Vertigo: light-headedness (10)
- Persistent frontal headache (8)
- Headaches
- Prominent eyeballs, painful eyes
- Optic neuritis (7)
- Great thirst for cold water (7)
- Nausea and car sickness (8)
- Delayed union of the fracture (7)
- Children: delayed development, undescended testicles (8)
- Hypertension, tachycardia
- Allergies: past or present
- Skin problems such as: dry, rough, itchy skin, psoriasis, eczema, urticaria, and angioedema
- Profuse sweat, moist palms

- Female: breast tumors, uterine fibroids
- All symptoms aggravated during pregnancy
- Enuresis in weak children who are nervous and irritable (8)

Aggravation

Worse: least exertion
Worse: heart symptoms worse by stooping or lying down
Worse: getting cold

Amelioration

Better: with contact
Better: motion (Rhus toxicodendron, Ruta graveolens)
Better: with rest

Causation

- Severe mental strain leading to diabetes
- History of sexual abuse or sexual indulgence
- Cretinism: severe hypothyroidism in an infant or child (the result of maternal iodine deficiency)
- Myxedema (advanced hypothyroidism when thyroid hormones are not being produced)

Contra-indications for Thyroidinum

Giving Thyroidinum during a fever is contra-indicated as it may deepen the pathology. When the fever is gone and Thyroidinum is given, the fever may return. Dr. Ghosh states, "It is therefore inadvisable to use it after the fever stops in acute infectious disease unless body economy is in a condition to develop proper immunity against a relapse." (26)

Thyroid Physiology

Hypothalamus

The hypothalamus is a small part of the brain that mediates the endocrine, autonomic, and behavior functions. The hypothalamus controls the release of hormones involved in temperature regulation, food and water intake, sexual behavior and reproduction, and mediation of emotional responses. (34) The Hypothalamus secretes TSH Releasing Hormone (TRH), which tells the pituitary gland to stimulate the thyroid gland to release TSH. (34)

Pituitary Gland

The pituitary gland is the master gland because it directs other organs and endocrine glands. As a master gland, the pituitary controls traffic, telling endocrine glands to induce or suppress hormone production. The pituitary gland is divided into the anterior and posterior lobes. The anterior pituitary regulates Thyrotropin-releasing hormone (TSH). (34)

Thyroid Gland

The thyroid gland is a part of the endocrine system. Two lobes are connected by an isthmus. The thyroid plays a vital role in regulating the body's metabolism and calcium balance.

The Thyroxine (T4) and Triiodothyronine (T3) hormones stimulate every tissue in the body to produce proteins and increase the amount of oxygen used by cells. The harder the cells work, the harder the organs work. The calcitonin hormone works together with the parathyroid hormone to regulate calcium levels in the body. (34)

Levels of hormones secreted by the thyroid are controlled by the pituitary gland: thyroid-stimulating hormone, which is governed by the hypothalamus. (34)

Tips for Thyroidinum

To understand the remedy Thyroidinum, it is valuable to know the most predominant hypothyroidism symptoms. Here is a helpful list:

- Tired, weak, fatigue
- Depression
- Impaired memory

- Anxiety, panic attacks (22, 23)
- Premenstrual syndrome: gas, bloating, weight gain, fluid retention, headaches, depression, irritability, fatigue, constipation, increase bruising, muscle aches (21, 23)
- Chilliness
- Dry skin
- Brittle nails
- Thinning hair
- Enlarged neck
- Constipation
- Weight gain
- Puffy face
- Hoarseness
- Muscle weakness
- Muscle aches: soreness and stiffness
- Pain: stiffness or swelling in the joints
- Heavier than normal or irregular menstrual periods
- Slow heart rate
- Elevated blood cholesterol level

Thyroidinum: The Forgotten Medicine

Until lately, Thyroidinum was the forgotten medicine in homeopathy. In 1998, Dr. Sarkar was granted a fellowship from the World Health Organization (WHO). During his fellowship, Dr. Sarkar introduced homeopathic Thyroidinum to the medical students at Southwest College of Naturopathic Medicine Health and Science, located in Tempe, Arizona.

When taking patients' cases, Dr. Sarkar was amazed by the clinical application of Thyroidinum in the college clinic. Thyroidinum stepped up to the front of the Materia Medica. He exclaimed, "The remedy has clear-cut applications and indications in the USA. Following keynotes and the patient's history, the application of the medicine changes lives. At times, this action is immediate and without side effects."

Dr. Sarkar was stunned at the difference between patients seen in India and Arizona. He stated over and over how clear-cut the keynotes were seen in female patients at the clinic, with a history of thyroid disease, a history of birth control use, and a craving for sweets. The medical students were amazed by his keen observation and explanations followed by the patients' results.

Dr. Sarkar comments, "Frankly, Thyroidinum may unlock deep cases where nothing seems to help." He echoed the thoughts of Dr. S.K. Ghosh, one of his favorite writers born in Kolkata, India. Dr. S.K. Ghosh stated, "This is a neglected medicine in Homeopathy. Seldom have Homeopaths taken services of this widely useful "Nosode." Particularly in cases with deep- seated chronic complications, it unlocks many a tangle and makes an easy way to cure." (27)

Let us take a deeper look at the thyroid pathology and keynotes for Thyroidinum. Memorizing and then recognizing the keynotes during a case will lead the homeopath to select this most important sarcode. In turn, the patient may turn around as Thyroidinum is one of our deepest medicines and cannot be replaced.

Dr. John Clarke, MD leaves us with a long list of clinical settings where Thyroidinum may be selected if the picture fits. These include a few that we usually would not think of using, including phthisis or tuberculosis and optic neuritis. (10)

Thyroidinum: A History of Birth Control Pills

Thyroidinum can be considered a remedy when there is a contraceptive pill history. TBG binds available thyroid hormones and therefore causes a decreased thyroid hormone level. Let us look at a list of common side effects of the birth control pill:

- Acne
- Breast tenderness and enlargement
- Breakthrough bleeding and spotting between periods
- Nausea and vomiting
- Changes in eye anatomy that makes it more difficult to wear contacts
- Headaches
- Bloating
- Weight gain
- Hirsutism or excessive hair growth
- Blood clots

- Mood swings
- Depression
- Migraines
- High blood pressure
- High cholesterol
- Allergic reactions such as rashes, hives, itching, swelling, and wheezing.
- Edema of the legs

Consider the hypothetical case of a Thyroidinum patient. This simulated narration or case may be helpful and is only for teaching purposes. Let us look at the life of "Dull Dora." One can easily see all the indications for prescribing Thyroidinum.

The Case of Dull Dora

Dora sits before us in a comfortable chair with a hoodie and boots, even in the California summer. Her hands are tucked into the pockets of her hoodie because they are cold. When you touch Dora's arms and hands, she feels cold. Her HANDS ARE COLD. She tells you she is chilly even in summer. The patient that requires Thyroidinum is CHILLY.

Dora's FEET ARE COLD. Even though it is summer, she has been wearing socks to bed. She loves boots with fake fur inside, even though it is summer, sweltering, and the temperature today is in the 90's in San Francisco Bay Area.

Dora has been checking her temperature and announces in a HOARSE VOICE that she has a daily, sub-normal temperature. She assures you she has checked her temperature first thing in the morning over many days. The results are the same; her temperature is always sub-normal.

As Dora continues with her narration of symptoms, she tells you she feels unrefreshed in the morning. She feels SLOW and SLUGGISH; maybe, she adds, it is due to her ongoing CONSTIPATION. She has tried everything for her constipation. Herbs, a high fiber diet, psyllium, and oils, such as flaxseed, fish oils, and even Castor oil, but nothing seems to help.

She explains due to her present history of constipation; she is quite IRRITABLE and short with just about everyone. She is embarrassed about her "new personality." She snaps at everyone and finds herself in a RAGE OVER THE LEAST LITTLE TRIFLE.

Most of all, she is discouraged about her recent WEIGHT GAIN. Just about any food makes her gain a pound or two. She is upset as she used to be the belle of the ball, but now her clothes are tight, and she has a feeling of DESPAIR.

She exclaims, "The pounds do not come off easily. My metabolism is slow, VERY SLOW. I am quite sure that my metabolism has come to a halt!"

Dora seems DEPRESSED about her health, mood, and weight gain. She states, "I am irritable, fed up, and discouraged about my whole life."

Dora tells you she has a very SWEET TOOTH. She constantly craves something sweet, which doesn't seem to help her weight. Sweets are always on her mind. As she has been so IRRITABLE lately, she now considers CHOCOLATE her best friend. Due to her irritability, she claims all her other friends have disappeared.

"When did all the symptoms begin?"

She explains, "Things have changed over the past two years or so. There was a gradual change; I cannot remember when all my new health issues began."

Dora is DISCOURAGED. She tells you this is her new life, "DULL DORA." She tells you she is as dull as a doorknob. She DESPAIRS OF RECOVERY.

Dora explains further, "Of course, somehow, I drag myself to work. I go through the motions, but I do not have any energy. Once I am at home alone, I have no energy. I DESIRE TO LAY DOWN and do nothing."

When you thought, as her physician, that you could take a deep breath, she tells you the worst is yet to come.

- She describes her CONSTANT MUSCLE ACHES AND WEAKNESS.
- She has ongoing HEADACHES.
- She explains that none of her health symptoms sense to her.

She is discouraged and cannot understand why other physicians she has seen cannot tell her what is wrong. "They run all sorts of laboratory tests and tell me I am fine. Other physicians tell me I just need more fresh air, eat less, and exercise. I guess I shall remain Dull Dora for the rest of my life."

Allergies, Hives, and Angioedema

The Thyroidinum Patient may tell you they have a long history of allergies that started in childhood. When eating the wrong food or something they are sensitive to, the patient develops allergic symptoms, such as a runny nose, conjunctivitis, hives, or angioedema. The patient will explain they have constant puffiness around their eyes. The angioedema may develop shortly after eating. Their face may swell quickly, which can be frightening.

Hives or urticaria is a constant problem for *The Thyroidinum Patient*, and usually they cannot guess the offending food or source of the hives.

- *The Thyroidinum Patient* selects their diet with care.
- Milk seems to be problematic.

- Wheat and other gluten-containing foods are a real problem.
- *The Thyroidinum Patient* avoids many foods and is better for the decision.

Here is a clue: When leading remedies such as Natrum muriaticum may be indicated, with bread and wheat intolerance but fail to act, think about the remedy Thyroidinum.

There may be a family history of allergies for *The Thyroidinum Patient*. Their mother, father, or even a grandparent may have a history of allergies. The patient may point out thyroid issues on one or both sides of the family. A family history of asthma may be present.

Thyroidinum can be thought of with angioedema in the history. At times angioedema is present at the change of seasons. Perhaps the patients will tell you that the angioedema is worse at each season's change. Your ears should perk up. Make sure to touch their palms and hand. If the skin is rough and dry, think about Thyroidinum. Remember, *The Thyroidinum Patient* is apt to be chilly.

Dr. Sarkar sums it all up, "*The Thyroidinum Patient* tells you their angioedema seems to be worse with the change of seasons. Their hives are worse with cold weather, cold, or seem to appear when they get angry. *The Thyroid Patient* finds that their hands are rough with the winter season, ROUGHER THAN NORMAL. Their skin is normally dry, but their skin is especially challenging in the winter. Remember, *The Thyroidinum Patient* is chilly. Their hands and feet are cold. *The Thyroidinum Patient* feels better with a warm application, warm weather, and worse when chilly."

Helpful Hints

- Angioedema: worse with the CHANGE OF SEASON
- Hives: worse with COLD WEATHER
- Hands: their skin is ROUGH
- Skin in the winter: Very DRY
- *The Thyroidinum Patient* is CHILLY
- They have COLD hands and feet

Dr. Sarkar continues, "Rashes are generally a headache for the doctor. Thyroidinum can be one of the most important remedies indicated. Listen to a patient who comes to you, telling you of constant rashes. With a rash that requires Thyroidinum, the rash is extreme. THINK BIG. THINK MORE! The Thyroidinum rash is more exaggerated in size and swelling."

Think big, Think more: Rashes, Urticaria, and Angioedema

- More **Edema** than one would see
- More **Swelling** than one would see
- More **Area** involved than one would see

- More **Itching** than burning than one would feel
- More **Heat** is better, as the Thyroidinum patient is CHILLY

Conjunctivitis

Conjunctivitis can be complicated or straightforward, but it is always thought-provoking for the doctor. There are four types of conjunctivitis, viral, bacterial, allergic, and conjunctivitis caused by a foreign body that irritates the eye tissue.

Physically the signs are often difficult to distinguish. Allergic conjunctivitis is usually bilateral but not always. Characteristic symptoms with bilateral allergic conjunctivitis produce watery discharge and can be accompanied by itching. The other conditions would probably start in one eye, the discharge would be thicker and stickier, and the pain would be more burning and stinging.

Eczema

Dr. S.K. Ghosh describes the history of eczema in *The Thyroidinum Patient* as overwhelming and difficult to describe due to the numerous manifestations it presents. (27) When skin symptoms are overwhelming for the patient, then think about Thyroidinum. This remedy is a gem and may come to the patient's rescue.

Complex Cases of Eczema

- **Local itching:** with eruptions, past treatment difficult
- **Rough skin:** palms, soles, and other areas
- **Edema:** redness, heat, swelling in the area
- **Itching in other areas:** nose, eyes, rectum
- **History of asthma:** in self or family members
- **History of food allergies:** there may be many, and patients have difficulty tracing the problematic foods

Allergies

Dr. Sarkar explains, "When thinking about recurrent allergies or prevention of allergies, we can employ, or think of the nosodes. Tuberculinum, Medorrhinum, and Psorinum are high on my list. Of course, Thyroidinum and Sulfur are our deep-acting remedies for allergies and cannot be forgotten. One can say that deeper acting remedies and nosodes must be introduced for chronic disease or tough cases. Allergies are tough to treat, and prevention is even more difficult. We must think deep and big. We must employ our deeper acting medicines for a difficult task."

Prevention of Recurrence of Allergies: Remedies to Consider:

- Medorrhinum
- Psorinum
- Sulfur

- Thyroidinum
- Tuberculinum

Fibrocystic Breast Disease: A Thyroidinum Example

The Thyroidinum Patient comes to you saying she developed fibrocystic breast disease when she began taking birth control contraceptive pills. She is chilly and tells you her hands and feet are cold even in the summer. She is glad to live in Arizona, where the temperature averages 105 degrees Fahrenheit in the summer, as it helps her warm up.

Her menses are her main problem as everything is aggravated before her menses. Her breasts are tender and painful. Before her menses, she craves sweets, chocolate, and anything that has an immense amount of sugar in it. She is flabby and states she has gained weight ever since she started using birth control pills. She has a history of food allergies and angioedema after taking medication and has felt puffy ever since.

The patient is shy, timid, and perhaps peevish, explaining that every small thing seems to upset her. She has difficulty telling you her story due to her introverted personality. She explains further that all her symptoms were even worse when she was pregnant. She had non-stop heartburn. At the time of pregnancy, she was unaware of a gluten allergy but realizes now the heartburn could have been prevented by a better diet void of bread and gluten-containing foods. She tells you that all her symptoms were worse during pregnancy. All she could do was think about creamy Swiss chocolate. Chocolate seemed to make her feel better and raise her spirits.

Optic Neuritis

Now let me address the elephant in the room. The elephant in the room is a patient who develops optic neuritis after receiving a vaccination or a set of vaccinations. The result is quite startling, especially if you are on the receiving end, as sudden blindness will quickly change one's life.

Optic neuritis is the swelling or inflammation of the optic nerve. The optic nerve consists of a bundle of fibers that provides visual information from the eye to the brain. The second cranial nerve involves vision. Optic neuritis usually affects one eye.

Mayo Clinic: Symptoms of Optic Neuritis

According to the Mayo Clinic, there are multiple symptoms, and they can vary from patient to patient. (27)

Pain. Most people who develop optic neuritis have eye pain that's worsened by eye movement. Sometimes the pain feels like a dull ache behind the eye.

Vision loss in one eye. Most people have at least some temporary reductions in vision, but the extent of loss varies. Noticeable vision loss usually develops over hours or days and improves over several weeks to months. Vision loss is permanent in some people.

Visual field loss. Side vision loss can occur in any pattern, such as central vision loss or peripheral vision loss.

Loss of color vision. Optic neuritis often affects color perception. Colors may appear less vivid than normal.

Flashing lights. Some people with optic neuritis report seeing flashing or flickering lights with eye movements.

Although neurological diseases with their vast symptoms are enough to get the hair up on one's back and cause the best Naturopathic physician or homeopathic doctor to have slight anxiety, one must remember good history taking is essential and the key to success.

Like any other case, following all the steps necessary to complete the case history will be essential. A complete case includes the family history. All the little food "likes and dislikes" may uncover a sweet tooth and a love of chocolate.

There can be much anxiety for the patient diagnosed with optic neuritis. As the one-sided blindness can be quite sudden, and the patient may feel extremely unwell.

A patient may find out they have a loss of vision at the ophthalmologist during an examination, as vision compensates when there is a loss, as the body tries to bring itself back into homeostasis.

The suddenness of the illness and the mere diagnosis shock may also bring on an episode of complete fear or despair of recovery.

As it takes time to heal from optic neuritis, the patient may feel depressed or worry about recovery. Allopathic medication given to the patient can save their vision but can have serious side effects.

Mind Symptoms of optic neuritis to remember:

- Anxiety
- Fear
- Depression
- Despair of recovery
- Irritation with the slightest little opposition

A Case of Optic Neuritis

The patient sitting in front of you developed optic neuritis quite suddenly in her left eye a year ago. When her vision returned after some months, she has been diagnosed with color blindness. She exhibits the following symptoms:

- She is chilly and has cold hands and feet.
- She has a history of constipation and feels slow and sluggish most of the time.
- The patient has a love of chocolate, claiming she must have a daily sampling.
- The patient is generally very thirsty and desires cold water or iced tea.
- Upon examination, you may notice her nails are dry and cracked.
- Her hands and feet feel cold to the touch.
- You uncover a family history of allergies.
- One special note is a history of food allergies and treatment for angioedema after taking allopathic medication.
- The patient has a history of an arrhythmia that started during her early teenage years. At the time, her blood tests showed a high T4 level, and she had severe palpitations. The Cardiologist told her that her high thyroid levels caused her palpitations, which have continued throughout her life.
- When asked about a history of vaccinations, the patient tells you she had a set of Hepatitis B vaccinations required to work in surgery.
- One surprising note is a history of car sickness.

All these unusual symptoms and a history of an arrhythmia that came on during adolescence may lead you confidently to the remedy Thyroidinum.

This is a perfect storm of symptoms and a call for Thyroidinum. This is a perfect case where the symptoms are all perfectly laid out.

The medical students in West Bengal, India, who are totally on top of their game, often shout when they have a perfect lineup of symptoms, *"The patient has read Allen's Keynotes."* It certainly made my day.

Keynotes to remember for Thyroidinum:

- Cold hands and feet
- Dry, cracked, brittle nails
- Desires sweets
- Constipation
- A history of angioedema
- Optic neuritis
- Great thirst for cold water
- Car sickness
- Tachycardia
- A history of Hepatitis B vaccinations preceding optic neuritis

A Note from Dr. Sarkar

Dr. Sarkar's private notebook is filled with clinical pearls and gems. One day, Dr. Sarkar made a copy of his notes for me, encouraging me to write more on Thyroidinum. He stated with a solemn face, "I have written my own Materia Medica, now you must write yours!"

Chapter 11
TORULA CEREVISIAE

A Nosode from fungus: Saccharomyces Cerevisiae, Yeast Plant

KEYNOTES

Mind Symptoms

- Mood: irritable, restless, and nervous
- Mood: worries and exhaustion from worrying

Physical Symptoms

- Torula is a sycotic remedy (Thuja occidentalis)
- Disturbance of digestion (sycotic symptom)
- Digestion poor
- Stomach sour
- Constipation
- Bad taste in the mouth
- Nausea
- Belching gas
- Gas in the stomach and abdomen after eating
- Soreness all over the abdomen
- Rumbling in the abdominal region
- Pains are shifting in the abdominal region
- Lots of flatulence
- Child appears to be full
- Thirsty

- Children with disturbed sleep
- Child: restless and restless legs while sleeping
- Headache, worse with constipation
- Sneezing and wheezing, especially if around bread being baked
- Nasal discharge
- Eczema
- Eruptions
- Recurrent boils in many places

Aggravation

Worse: baking bread (Lycopodium)
Worse: when constipated (opposite of Calcarea carbonica)
Worse: sneezing and wheezing
Worse: from dust of any kind
Worse: at full moon
Worse: after a bath, the patient does not feel clean
Worse: going to sleep with an empty stomach
Worse: with expiration
Worse: breathing hard

Causation

- Gonorrhea or family history of gonorrhea
- Reactions from the protein in vaccinations:

    - Egg protein
    - Vero: monkey kidney cells
    - Calf serum
    - Bovine extract
    - Bovine casein

Dose:

- In the potentized form
- Dr. William Boericke states the dose can be given in "Pure yeast cakes or potencies from 3rd to higher ones."
- I have not baked the Pure Yeast Cakes myself. One must consider many patients have antibodies against Torula or nutritional yeast, therefor consider the homeopathic remedy.
- Anaphylactic states are produced by proteins and enzymes (Yingling)
- Dr. Sarkar uses Torula cerevisiae in potentized form. Of course!

The Nutritional Yeast Known as Brewer's Yeast

Torula or Saccharomyces cerevisiae is a yeast species well known and has been used since ancient times in baking and brewing. Torula reproduces by a division known as budding and is the primary source of nutritional yeast and yeast extract. (34)

Most interesting, "Antibodies against S. cerevisiae are found in 60–70% of patients with Crohn's disease and 10–15% of patients with Ulcerative colitis." (34)

According to Wikipedia, "Saccharomyces" derives from Latinized Greek and means "sugar mold" or "sugar fungus," saccharo- being the combining from "sugar-" and myces being "fungus." Cerevisiae comes from Latin and means "of beer." (35)

Other names for Torula or Saccharomyces cerevisiae are: (35)

- S. cerevisiae: a short form of the scientific name
- Brewer's yeast
- Ale yeast
- Top-fermenting yeast
- Baker's yeast
- Budding yeast

Homeopathic Materia Medica

Dr. Sarkar states with conviction, "We must consider Torula cerevisiae when a child or an adult has had a bad effect from vaccination. It is a real gem, and each child with disabilities, whether mental or physical, where there is a link to vaccinations, must be prescribed Torula. To date, it may be our most important remedy."

Torula addresses the anaphylactic state produced by a protein, such as chicken eggs, or enzymes from the vaccination directly. Torula is perhaps one of the most important remedies for a child on the autism spectrum. It will undoubtedly address mind symptoms, such as restlessness, nervousness, and anxiety.

Digestive symptoms, rumbling, constipation, and abdominal tenderness are the main keynotes for Torula. We must not forget distress, discomfort, and constipation are the key symptoms that keep the child from healing. The healing takes place in both body and mind with Torula.

There is no doubt that Torula is one of our leading remedies for this point and time in history. This remedy is amazing for children, especially when there is a history of gonorrhea in the family history. Don't forget that Torula has a sycotic origin, and thus we will see severe symptoms in the child.

Let us break down the keynotes one by one so the prescriber can understand and compare Materia Medica. It is essential to know single remedies, their keynotes and not partake in the application of multi-remedies. A cookbook approach is not the best approach.

Case Example

Yesterday, a child with autism entered my clinic after having been seen by two top-notch homeopaths who were also pediatricians. The first pediatrician had the patient on a multitude of combination remedies. The second pediatrician added more. All in total, the best I could figure out, the child was taking 90 remedies!

The mother was worried about the child's health, as he was soon to have a tonsillectomy. She did not want the child to get sick before his surgery. The pediatrician added another combo remedy to keep the child well. There were 12 remedies combined in that bottle which meant the child would have been taking 102 remedies daily. When hearing the news that the child was receiving over 100 remedies all at once, I was alarmed. How does one deal with such a situation? I ask, "Do you treat the patient *and* the doctor in this case?"

My immediate questions were, "What remedy is doing what? Who would know if there was a proving with so many daily remedies? And then: "Who would be able to sort out the proving symptoms? Which remedy did they come from?"

I do not know anyone who has the answer to these questions. I have asked Dr. Sarkar to comment many times on the subject of multi-remedies. He was stunned by my question and stated, "There is no answer. Nobody knows when there is a series of combination remedies given to a child. One thing for sure I do advise: Learn Materia Medica and give a proper prescription based on the proving, keynotes and information left by the masters. Pour your whole heart and mind into your work. Learn the remedies one by one. It may take years for this kind of knowledge. Dedication to one's life work is important! It is a must."

When I looked at the boxes of multi-remedies, all I could think of was Dr. H.C. Allen's Keynotes and Characteristics located under the remedy Staphysagria, "Great indignation about things done by others or himself; grieves about the consequences." I will leave my precious keynote at that and save further discussion. However, I shall take one dose of Staphysagria for my suppressed feelings about the use of multiple remedies given at the same time and use prayer for the child's sake!

It is six years later, and the child is doing well. He excels in his studies. During his initial appointment, I had a heart-to-heart with the mother. She threw out all the multi-remedies. One remedy, Veratrum album, was prescribed, and the following month the child was much better on every account.

Irritability and Nervousness Is the Key

Torula cerevisiae paints the perfect picture of a child with autism. The child is irritable and cranky. The child is nervous, and every little change makes the situation worse. During their interview, a parent will quickly state that the child is worse with transitions. The child worries about every little trifle and appears wholly worn out from his worries. *The Torula Child* has no energy left over for learning.

The Torula Child's irritability is seen in remedies such as Cina and Chamomilla. Cina and Chamomilla are both better being carried. Cina is tough to calm down. *The Cina Child* can be found screaming on the floor in my clinic, striking anyone that comes near or touches him. When in a rage, *The Chamomilla Child* will also strike out at anyone near him.

Take a good history and look at the keynotes. At times, I find the remedies' choice is in the modalities. Torula is worse after a bath, during a full moon, and going to bed hungry. These modalities may help. Now, it is up to you to decide between the remedies.

Brain-Gut Connection

Research shows a direct connection between the brain and the gastrointestinal system. The child that requires Torula may present with gas, abdominal distension, flatulence, and constipation. The child's irregular digestion and eating habits may be due to nausea, severe constipation, or both.

The child may have a sense of fullness, causing symptoms such as a sore abdomen that is sensitive to touch. These symptoms may lead to sluggishness often seen in a child with autism. The child may not want to talk, play, or learn their ABC's. The child may have additional symptoms such as emotional irritability and nervousness.

This picture is a close resemblance of Bryonia alba, and you must pick between the two. Both remedies are thirsty with little desire to work. They share many keynotes, such as irritability, headaches, and severe constipation. Bryonia is better still and dislikes to be carried. Torula is restless. I leave you with these thoughts.

Comparative Materia Medica: Constipation

With homeopathy, the doctor must continuously think about Comparative Materia Medica for the sake of the patient. Comparison between the remedies is essential. Knowledge of the individual remedies selected for the bad effects of vaccinations can really make a difference in healing and the progress of the child. Therefore, a comparison must be made between Torula cerevisiae and Calcarea carbonica.

Constipation seen in a child that requires Torula is different, or has a different, presentation than a child who needs Calcarea carbonica. The parents know something is wrong with the child's digestion.

- *The Torula Child* feels full.
- *The Torula Child* is uncomfortable.
- The child's abdomen is sensitive to touch.
- The child has gas, lots of gas, and flatulence.
- *The Torula Child* burps.
- *The Torula Child* has pain in their abdomen, and the pains seem to shift.
- The child has lots of wind but no poop.
- Constipation makes the child irritable and fussy.
- *The Torula Child* is nervous and fearful.

It is not so with Calcarea carbonica. In fact, it is quite the opposite. Sure, Calcarea carbonica is constipated, but they don't have all the fuss and bother about being constipated. Here is the clue; Calcarea carbonica feels better when constipated.

Dr. H.C. Allen leads us right to the keynote, "Feels better in every way when constipated." This one line, this short keynote, will make the difference as both are chilly remedies and have cold hands.

Burping

The Torula Child is nauseated and may burp continuously. In comparison, Carbo vegetabilis has powerful keynotes that are seen frequently.

Keynotes to remember for Carbo vegetabilis:

- Eructation, worse after eating
- Temporarily better after burping
- Burping, better burping
- Burping gives temporary relief
- Child: distended abdomen

As Dr. E.B. Nash would say, "I have given you all the clues; you must choose between the two."

In Summary:

- When thinking about Torula cerevisiae, many remedies come to mind.
- Torula has the irritability of Cina, Chamomilla, and Bryonia.

- Constipation and chilliness of Calcarea carbonica are present.
- Torula has the burping of Carbo vegetabilis.
- *The Torula Child* is irritable, has constipation, headaches, and the thirst of Bryonia.

When seeing a picture with such a grand statement or keynotes in a child with many gastrointestinal symptoms after vaccinations, think Torula cerevisiae.

- **Irritability:** of Chamomilla and Cina
- **Constipation and chilliness:** of Calcarea carbonica
- **Irritability, constipation, and thirst:** of Bryonia alba
- **Burping:** of Carbo vegetabilis

Chapter 12
VACCININUM

A Nosode from Vaccine Matter: Lymph of Cowpox

KEYNOTES

Mind Symptoms

- Child wants to be carried (26)
- Impatient and irritable (7)
- Crying, ill humor (7)
- Ill-humored with restless sleep (7)
- Morbid fear of taking the smallpox vaccine (7)
- Easily troubled (7)
- Tired all over, with stretching, gaping feeling (wide open feeling)
- Unnatural fatigue (26)
- Weakness (7)
- Restlessness, malaise, weakness after vaccination (26)
- Nervous depression, impatient, irritable (7)
- Confusion: she does not remember things when she wants them (7)
- Patient faints when being vaccinated (26)

Physical Symptoms

- Small pimples develop at the point of vaccination with the fourth dilution (7)

- Keratitis after vaccination (26)
- Nephritis and albuminuria, hematuria and dropsy developed eleven days or soon after vaccination; child recovered (26)
- Severe pains in left upper arm at vaccination mark, could not raise arm in the morning (26)
- Cheloids on re-vaccination marks (26)
- Redness on the left upper arm
- A general eruption similar to cowpox (7)

Aggravation

- The worse time of the day is morning (Burnett)

Peculiar Sensations of Vaccininum

- As if forehead were split
- As if the bones of the leg were broken and undergoing a process of comminution (broken into pieces)
- As if flying in the air
- As if eyes would be pierced from within outward
- As if a thread were hanging from the throat downward

Introduction

The remedy Vaccininum is made from the lymph of cowpox; therefore, Vaccininum is considered a nosode. Dr. Fincke and Dr. Swan carried out the original provings of this remedy.

Can we toss this remedy aside, considering the vaccination for smallpox is not made from cowpox anymore? As Dr. E.B. Nash uses the term, one must "Study up!" And I had to study up to answer my question. I knew the answer, but I needed proof as my reader may be skeptical.

"The proof of the pudding" is in the eating! It's an ancient proverb that teaches us:

- Learn the history of the remedy Vaccininum
- Listen to the patient
- Look at the details of the case
- Compare the symptoms to the remedy
- Are the symptoms strange or rare?

Dr. John Clarke, MD made a list of clinical uses to think about using homeopathy principles when considering Vaccininum. Here is the list:

- Cheloid, eczema, leprosy
- Naevus, nephritis, smallpox
- Tumors, vaccinia, vaccinosis
- Whooping cough

Dr. William Boericke gives us a little more information in his introduction of Vaccininum, "Vaccine poison is capable of setting up a morbid state of extreme chronicity, named after Burnett Vaccinosis; symptoms are like those of Hahnemann's sycosis."

Dr. Boericke goes further with a broad description of symptoms, "Neuralgias, inverterate skin eruptions, chilliness, indigestion with great flatulent distension (Clarke). Whooping cough."

"Boericke is quite short and stingy with the rest of his Materia Media on this subject," as only Dr. Sarkar, a scholar in Materia Medica, would be bold enough to state! However, a short note under the title *Relationship* that is important: Boericke writes 'Compare: anti-vaccinal remedies; Variolinum, Malandrinum, Thuja. Powerful Adjuvants in the Treatment of Malignant Disease.'"

The last part of the statement might be helpful for homeopaths that specialize in oncology. On the note of cancer, there is an exciting point to compare under Malandrinum, "Efficacious in the clearing of the remnants of cancerous deposits (Cooper)." Food for thought and maybe action.

Under Characteristics in Dr. Clarke's: *A Dictionary of Practical Materia Medica*, we find the juice, the nuts and bolts, the helpful tidbits that aid us in understanding the remedy, history, and application of this nosode.

"Vaccinia, Smallpox, and Grease of the horse are inter-related diseases, and the nosode of each are available for the treatment and prevention of all three. Vaccine poison can set up a morbid state of extreme chronicity, named after Burnett Vaccinosis. And it may do this without causing the primary symptoms: when the vaccination does not take. The symptoms of vaccinosis are protean and are, for the most part, identical with the symptoms of Sycosis of Hahnemann. Vaccinosis which is a sycotic disease."

Dr. H.C. Allen states, "Vaccininum 200th quickly severs symptoms of variola occurring in a child, age, six months; two days before the appearance of the eruption had been re-vaccinated (after an interval of eight days) on a nevus near right nipple; deglutition difficult through implication of tongue and fauces; pustules, many of large size, scattered over the scalp, face, body, and limbs." (7)

Dr. S. K. Ghosh, of Kolkata states, "Treated a great many cases of variola and varioloid during last eighteen years, some of them of the most desperate character, and yet never lost a case when employing vaccine virus as a remedy; moreover, none of the cases so treated were ever troubled with hemorrhage, or with delirium, or secondary fevers, or were ever disfigured with pitting." (26)

Ill-Humored and Restless

With Vaccininum, we see an upset, irritable, angry child that has just been vaccinated. The child is ill-humored. He wants to be carried. He is easily upset, flying off the handle and losing his temper. In this way, we can compare the mind symptoms of Vaccininum with Chamomilla and Cina.

With Vaccininum, more symptoms may manifest. The child is exhausted but restless at the same time. When the child does sleep, he is restless.

Skin Irritation

Vaccininum is predominantly a left-sided remedy due to vaccinations given on the left side of the body. If there is a history of smallpox re-vaccination, this remedy is called for upon seeing cheloid formation. If vaccinated on the left arm, the child will present with redness.

The skin appears hot and dry. Red pimples, blotchy skin, and eruptions of pustules can be seen. The skin symptoms are mainly on the left side, affecting the left arm and shoulder, but the eruptions may cover the whole body.

Dr. H. C. Allen describes the eruptions that are similar to cowpox. "Small pimples develop at the point of vaccination with fourth dilution." (26)

Whooping Cough

Dr. John Clarke, MD leaves us with a significant case, "Some years ago an old-school observer vaccinated for some reason a child whilst suffering from whooping cough, and whooping cough vanished. He repeated the experiment in other cases, and with such signal success that he wrote to the journals recommending it as a routine practice in the case of unvaccinated children. On the other hand, homeopathic observers have seen whooping cough follows immediately on vaccination and have cured with Thuja." (30)

We have a lot to digest and then put into practice considering this last statement, as whooping cough is still prevalent. Drosera rotundifolia and Thuja can be compared with Vaccininum.

Drosera has an important keynote that may lead the way. "Whooping cough with violent paroxysms which follows each other rapidly, scarcely able to get breath (wakes at 6-7 a.m. and does not cease coughing until a large quantity of tenacious mucus is raised.)" (26)

I have had many cases of whooping cough in my practice. Upon watching and listening to a child or adult coughing, I have sharpened my hearing and have memorized the deep-sounding, rapid cough followed by a high-pitched "whoop" sound.

I have been in the practice of giving Drosera based on keynotes. Drosera has in my practice relieved the patient, who is exhausted from coughing, and given them hope. The effect has been immediate. The best writings I have found on Drosera are by Dr. M. L. Tyler in her textbook *Homoeopathic Drug Pictures*. I have used Drosera 200C potency in my practice.

Just an interesting note, about five years ago, a whole family was vaccinated for Tetanus, Diphtheria, and Pertussis in autumn. Public Health Officials strongly advised them to vaccinate as the mother was pregnant and a new baby was on the way. The family did choose to vaccinate, knowing that whooping cough is a deadly disease for infants.

In January, the whole family was diagnosed with whooping cough, including the baby. I gave all six of them the homeopathic remedy that fit their symptoms best, according to the keynotes written clearly by Dr. H.C. Allen. Drosera made them immediately feel better, and their cough decreased immediately. The baby did well and had a very mild case of whooping cough.

During the 2014 winter, I treated many patients, with great success, with whooping cough. As Naturopathic physicians, or homeopathic doctors, we must be prepared and know our signs and symptoms of the disease and keynotes. Materia Medica's knowledge is the ticket, and when the proper remedy is applied, our patients' sufferings will be minimal.

Pertussis or whooping cough historically recurs every three to five years. In California, the last outbreak was in 2014. According to reports from the California Department of Public Health, 11,000 cases were reported, and two infants died.

Bad Effects of Vaccination

According to the WHO, smallpox has been globally eradicated; we should not forget its history and what the vaccination for smallpox has done to save mankind.

According to Wikipedia, "During the 20th century, it is estimated that smallpox was responsible for 300-500 million deaths." Even though smallpox has been eradicated, there are still patients with a history of smallpox, symptoms that are the sequelae of smallpox, and horrible scars that remind the doctor of this disease and the hurricane history it has left us in; its wake." (28)

The most modern application of the remedy Vaccininum comes from Dr. Sarkar. He gives background information about the here and now and the fact that Vaccininum has been long forgotten, misunderstood, and pushed aside.

Dr. Sarkar explains: "Vaccininum is an important remedy and should be on the list of, *Do Not Forget Remedies*, instead of *Long Forgotten Remedies!* And since I am on a roll, let me tell you more. Vaccininum is an important remedy when there are bad effects from a vaccination. This clinically is most important for the children that suffer from vaccination effects where allopathic medicine has no answers nor help for the child. In this case, Torula cerevisiae or Saccharomyces cerevisiae can be followed with Vaccininum. Although it is a little cookbook secret of mine, I am more than willing to share the knowledge I have for the sake of humanity."

"Now, after saying my thoughts, that are really my worries, I shall add on to this intense study of Vaccininum. I use Vaccininum frequently in my practice, as Dr. Tarasuk knows well and has reminded me. When a patient comes in with scars left from smallpox, we must think of this remedy."

Studying with a great master of homeopathy throughout the years has educated me in many ways. Working alongside Dr. Sarkar year after year in a village on the outskirts of Kolkata has broadened my skill set as a physician. Seeing an unbelievable number of patients daily in his clinic has introduced me to tropical diseases and sequela of diseases such as smallpox that I have not seen in California. Using modern diagnostic tools such as blood tests, MRI, X-rays, and ultrasounds to diagnose and follow up demonstrates how solid and reliable homeopathy treatments are.

We must not forget or put aside remedies like Vaccininum. Following keynotes, signs, and symptoms of the patient can lead us to the treatment if we use the principle of homeopathy. With a bit of studying, Vaccininum will come to the forefront again. However, we must never forget smallpox and the suffering of humanity. Knowing the signs and symptoms of the disease and the history sharpens our minds and helps with the clinical application of Vaccininum.

End Notes

1. Harnischfeger G, Stolze H. Bewährte *Pflanzendrogen in Wissenschaft und Medizin*. Notamed Verlag, Bad Homburg/ Melsungen; 1983. pp. 250–9.

2. Witte l, Berlin J, Wray V, Schubert W, Kohl W, Höfle G, Hammer J. Mono- und diterpenes from cell cultures of *Thuja occidentalis*. Planta Med. 1983, Volume 49, pp. 216–21. https://pubmed.ncbi.nlm.nih.gov/17405056/

3. Brijesh K, Ruchi R, Das S, Phytoconstituents and Therapeutic potential of Thuja occidentalis. Research Journal of Pharmaceutical, Biological and Chemical Sciences. April – June 2012 RJPBCS Volume 3, Issue 2, p. 354.

4. UK Tea and Infusions Association, November 6, 2014. http://www.tea.co.uk/the-london-tea-auction

5. Clarke, J. *Clark Constitutional Medicine* with special reference to The Three Constitutions of Dr. Von Grauvogl. Presented by MédiT.
http://www.homeoint.org/books5/clarkeconstit/

6. "Glabella." *Wikipedia, The Free Encyclopedia*. November 13, 2013. Wikimedia Foundation, Inc. Web. Jan. 1, 2014.

7. Allen, Henry C. *Allen's Keynotes and Characteristics with Comparisons of Some of the Leading Remedies of the Materia Medica with Nosodes*. Reprint edition. New Delhi: B. Jain Publishers Pvt. Ltd., 2000.

8. Boericke, William. *New Manual of Homeopathic Materia Medica & Repertory*. Revised & Up-Dated edition. New Delhi: B. Jain Publishers Pvt. Ltd., 1999.

9. Cazalet, Sylvian. "Kent H.I." *Homeopathe International*. 2004. July 1, 2012.

10. Clarke, John H. *Dictionary of Practical Materia Medica Vol I-III*. Reprint Edition. New Delhi: B. Jain Publishers Pvt. Ltd., 1995.

11. Hering, Constantine. *The Guiding Symptoms of our Materia Medica Vol. I-IX*. Reprint edition. New Delhi: B. Jain Publishers Pvt. Ltd., 1997.

12. Kent, James T. *Repertory of The Homoeopathic Materia Medica And A Word Index*. Reprint edition. New Delhi: B. Jain Publishers Pvt. Ltd., 1995.

13. Nash, Eugene B. *Leaders in Homoeopathic Therapeutics*. Reprint edition. New Delhi: B. Jain Publishers Pvt. Ltd., 1997.

14. Schroyens, Frederik. *Synthesis: Repertorium Homeopathicum Syntheticum*. The Source Repertory. Edition 9.1. New Delhi: B. Jain Publishers Pvt. Ltd., 2004.

15. Schroyens, Frederik. *Synthesis: Repertorium Homeopathicum Syntheticum* 9.1 edition. New Delhi: B. Jain Publishers Pvt. Ltd., 2004.

16. Vermeulen, Frans. *Synoptic Materia Medica 2 the Complement to Prisma*. Third edition. Haarlem: Emryss bv Publishers, 2003.

17. Schroyens, Frederik. *1001 Small Remedies*. First edition. London: Homeopathic Book Publishers and Archibel S.A., 1995.

18. Kranowitz, C. S. *The Out-of-Sync Child Recognizing and Coping with Sensory Integration Dysfunction.* First edition. New York: Skylight Press, The Berkley Publishing Group, 1998.

19. Boger, C.M. *A Synoptic Key to The Materia Medica (A Treatise for Homoeopathic Students)* Reprint edition. New Delhi: B. Jain Publishers Pvt. Ltd., 1995.

20. Vithoulkas, G., Causation Cases and Cases with no Essence, Whole Health Now, 2014.
http://www.wholehealthnow.com/homeopathy_pro/

21. Kent, James T. *Lectures on Homoeopathic Philosophy.* Reprint edition. Berkley: North Atlantic Books, 1997.

22. Burnett, James. C., *Vaccinosis and Its Cure by Thuja with Remarks on Homeoprophylaxis.* Reprint edition. New Delhi: B. Jain Publishers Pvt. Ltd., 2006.

23. Margery Grace Blackie 1898-1981. Sue Young Histories Biographies of Homeopaths 2015.
http://sueyounghistories.com/archives/2008/08/07/margery-grace-blackie-and-homeopathy

24. Tyler, M.L., *Homoeopathic Drug Pictures* Reprint edition. New Delhi: B. Jain Publishers Pvt. Ltd., 1995.

25. Allen, Henry C. *The Materia Medica of the Nosodes with Provings of the X-Ray.* Reprint edition. New Delhi: B. Jain Publishers Pvt. Ltd., 2007.

26. Ghosh S. K. *Clinical Experience with Some Rare Nosodes.* Calcutta: Sm. Sushama Rani Ghosh., pp. 1-108, 1972.

27. Mayo Clinic, 2021. https://www.mayoclinic.org/diseases-conditions/optic-neuritis/symptoms-causes/syc-20354953

28. Wikipedia contributors. Smallpox. *Wikipedia, The Free Encyclopedia*. https://en.wikipedia.org/w/index.php?title=Smallpox&oldid=1016579703
https://En.Wikipedia.Org/Wiki/Smallpox

29. Walker, L.J., Anti-*Saccharomyces cerevisiae* antibodies (ASCA) in Crohn's disease are associated with disease severity but not NOD2/CARD15 mutations. Clinical and Experimental Immunology, 2004 Mar; 135(3): pp. 490–496. https://www.ncbi.nlm.nih.gov/pmc/articles/PMC1808965/

30. Pulford, A. *Homoeopathic Materia Medica of Graphic Drug Pictures and Clinical Comments*. Pulford, 1944.

31. Twain, M. (1897). *Following the Equator*. American Publishing Company Doubleday & McClure.

32. Wikipedia contributors. Mud Fever. *Wikipedia, The Free Encyclopedia*. Accessed April 2021 18:33 UTC, 2021. https://en.wikipedia.org/w/index.php?title=Mud_fever&oldid=996403168

33. Wikipedia contributors. Saccharomyces cerevisiae. *Wikipedia, The Free Encyclopedia*. Accessed 8 April 2021 18:15 UTC, 2021.
https://en.wikipedia.org/wiki/Saccharomyces_cerevisiae.

34. Wikipedia contributors. Thyroid. *Wikipedia, The Free Encyclopedia*. Accessed 4-10-2021, 2021.
https://en.wikipedia.org/w/index.php?title=Thyroid&oldid=1011125969

Acknowledgements

Dr. Janis Gruska, ND, Associate Academic and Clinical Professor, at Bastyr University reviewed this pocket guide. With her expertise in homeopathy and botanical medicine, she encouraged me to publish my pocket guide without further ado. Her words are always encouraging, her advice is spectacular, and her friendship is most valuable! Thank you!

My husband is to be commended once again. Matthew edits my work, although he admits, all these keynotes and Comparative Materia Medica are enough to put him to sleep. He is always willing, nevertheless. Matthew is my best friend.

Dr. Ann Seipt, ND tells me to keep on writing, teaching, and publishing. She is the best support and always tells me to "keep on keeping on." She has phoned weekly during the Covid-19 pandemic, telling me to stay home as I have to help others, my patients, and to think of the future. Dr. Seipt is kind and always thinks of the big picture. She is a great homeopath.

My son Dane is my best editor and a whiz at formatting. Where would I be without him? Writing and publishing a book is a family affair, where everyone is involved!

I want to thank my dear friend Dr. Himanshu Asani, PhD, winner of the Marconi Society Paul Baran Young Scholar Award, and Assistant Professor at School of Technology and Computer Science Tata Institute of Fundamental Research. We spent many hours talking about science, math, cancer, and homeopathy. Best friends share their knowledge and teach. Himanshu is an outstanding teacher.

Of course, where would I be without fabulous teachers that have taught me the clinical application of medicine and pathology, my second favorite subject? While in medical school Dr. Scott Luper, ND gave me unbelievable support and has continued with his clinical advice and deep friendship.

A big thank you also goes to Heather Carmichael, the Clinic Director at Southwest College of Naturopathic Medicine from 1997 to 2000, and head of the acupuncture program. In medical school, my professors treated me as a seasoned doctor way before my time. Heather continues to encourage me and has always been available with a smile. She is just a phone call away. I am glad to call her my friend.

I spent many hours in Dr. Sarkar's clinic, in West Bengal, India in what I call the jungle. We serviced many patients per day, with or without electricity, during "Monsoon Season," and at times, with the rain pouring down so heavily, I could not hear myself think.

In the early morning, over many "Monsoon Seasons," with the mosquitoes biting my feet, and through my clothes, I learned pathology and saw many diseases I had read about only in textbooks. If you have a sense of adventure, if you want to learn and see pathology, go to India.

I have had the opportunity to lecture in India and would like to thank the National Institute of Homeopathy that is under the Ministry of Ayurveda, Yoga & Naturopathy, Unani, Siddha, and Homeopathy, Government of India. Lecturing to the students in the grand assembly was exciting.

Lecturing to residents on autism at D.N. De Homoeopathic Medical College & Hospital, one of the oldest homeopathic medical colleges in Kolkata, West Bengal, India, was an honor. Lecturing in India is always a super experience that creates great memories which last forever. I have learned without a doubt that the West Bengal residents are brilliant and dedicated beyond belief.

Finally, I would like to thank Mother India, the patients who have taught me medicine, and the application of Ayurveda and Homeopathy. Without the love, kindness, and compassion of the people in West Bengal, these remedies would not be written.

Index To Remedies

About The Author

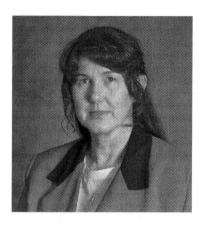

Denise Tarasuk is an international lecturer and a board-certified Naturopathic doctor specializing in homeopathic medicine. Her new release, *Pocket Guide: Homeopathic First Aid for Vaccinosis* is a timely and critical response to the global dilemma of vaccinosis, especially among children. Here are the 12 foremost remedies with keynotes, clinical tips and comparative Materia Medica from the legacy of the Grand Masters.

Printed in the United States
by Baker & Taylor Publisher Services